Erectile Dysfunction

What Worked for Us

By Jacob and Michelle Clark

FOREWARD
By Darrell Maloney, Author

I've known Jacob and Michelle for over half my life. Jacob was in the Army stationed in Kaiserslautern, West Germany, when I was in the Air Force stationed at nearby Spangdahlem.

Yes, I said "West Germany". In those days the country was still divided. We were lucky enough to be there when the wall came down in 1989.

Sometimes Army and Air Force people don't mix well. They're frequently like oil and water. But our two families were neighbors in the town of Wittlich and became fast friends.

When they asked me to write the foreward to their new book I jumped at the chance. You see, I got an early look at it and knew it was going to be a best seller someday.

The book is a bit gritty and frank sometimes. But then again, it's talking about a very serious subject.

Despite that, the authors managed to make it very entertaining as well as informative. It's roughly equal parts humor and serious advice. And chock full of little tidbits I never would have thought of.

But which may well help you conquer what they call "the ED monster."

I'm going on record here and now by saying this book will soon be the go-to "Bible" for every couple suffering the effects of erectile dysfunction.

Yes, it's that good.

Enjoy.

OKAY, WHERE DO WE START?

Erectile dysfunction continues to be a very personal and very troubling crisis.

It shouldn't be. For it's as normal as any other medical condition.

We wouldn't be ashamed because we were stricken with migraine headaches or varicose veins. Yet men are generally ashamed when stricken with the inability to obtain and maintain an erection. We feel as though we're somewhat les of a man than we once were. Like our virility has left our lives forever.

And even worse, we feel as though we've let our loved one down.

It doesn't have to be that way.

For all three of those things: the migraines, the varicose veins and the erectile dysfunction, are all perfectly normal, and treatable in a variety of ways.

We need to stop being stigmatized by a condition which occasionally strikes half of men over age forty five. Seventy six percent of men over sixty.

It's perfectly normal. And while we shouldn't embrace it as we would our best friend, we should stop being ashamed of it.

Rather, we should expect it and have a course of action ready when it strikes, so we can deal with it.

We need to get over our hesitancy to talk about it. Our doctors can't help us if they don't know about it.

Neither can our wives or girlfriends.

They are our best allies when it comes to dealing with this problem.

The good news… most of us can be "fixed," with a little tender loving care and patience from our spouses, and a willingness to be open and honest about our problem.

And... a willingness to try a variety of methods of dealing with ED until we find one that works.

That's the whole premise behind this book.

We (and we use that term because we considered it a problem to solve for both of us) have actually been there. We went through all the emotions, the frustration, the anger, the humiliation. We could have just given up on our sex life as so many people resign themselves to do.

But we didn't. Quite honestly, the "sex thing," as we playfully started calling it long ago, was too big a part of our lives. We had too much fun doing it. Our sex life was wide-ranging and fun.

And it felt amazingly good.

It wasn't something we wanted to give up.

But we've always been frank and honest with one another. It's been the cornerstone of our relationship since day one.

Jacob's difficulty in having and maintaining an erection was causing us problems. We couldn't deny it. It was depriving us of one of the most intimate and personal pleasures a man and a woman can share.

So we spoke about it... and we decided to treat it as we had every other problem we'd faced in our marriage. We were going at it together, as a team, and we were going to fight it and win.

Erectile dysfunction, commonly known as ED, was a formidable opponent.

And truth be known we know the battle may not be over with. That it could rear its very ugly head again at a later date.

But for the time being, we beat it.

And for the time being, we're celebrating by enjoying a very active sex life.

Not as active as we did in our twenties, but that's okay. Back then our bodies were younger and in better shape, and could handle the physical stress of rolling around on the bed (and the floor, and the kitchen counters) for hours on end and still get up and go to work the next day.

No, our sex life isn't like that, but then again it shouldn't be.

These days, every two or three nights, one or both of us get the urge to be intimate.

And these days, Jacob's body responds the way it once did, back in those days.

And it's nice. For both of us.

This book is about our journey, from the early days when ED decided to take away something near and dear to us, to the time we decided to fight back, and then the various things we did to combat it.

This book will be frank, and will occasionally use frank language and details. But it should be frank, because we're dealing with a very serious matter.

This book will provide you the reader some insight.

And perhaps some new ideas.

No one thing works for everyone. We all know that. But we'll discuss the things that worked for us, with the hope you'll be willing to try some of them yourselves.

Perhaps you can banish that ugly monster from your lives and send him packing as we did.

Perhaps you too can, as we did, take your sex life back and go at it with a ferocity you thought was gone forever.

The premise of this book is a simple one.

There are an awful lot of tools and techniques available to help you combat your ED problem.

Some work very well for some or most, but not at all for others.

Some work very poorly for most, but very well for just a few.

Some you've likely never even heard of.

Some perhaps you've heard of, but never thought to try.

We're going to educate you so you know which tools are out there.

We're going to open your mind and get you to consider all the tools available.

We're all different. The trick is to consider all the tools, and to find the tools which will work best for you. They may not be the same tools that work for the next guy, or the ones which worked for us.

But they're out there. If you keep an open mind and are willing to try the things we'll discuss, we're confident we can help.

FIRST, A LITTLE BIT ABOUT US...

From Jacob:

I'm fifty eight years old. I've been fascinated with the human mind for as long as I can remember. Specifically the way it controls and interacts with us physiologically. How the body and the mind work together to help us deal with things.

I've always been a passionate person. I was a boy who saved my pennies and my nickels, and who went out and got a paper route when I was twelve. Not because I was necessarily an ambitious young man.

No, rather because I needed the money. My family was rather poor, you see, and giving their children money for an allowance wasn't something my parents were willing to do. If I wanted money, I had to earn it.

But I didn't want it for the same things my friends did. I didn't go to the little convenience store on the corner to buy a bottle of soda or a candy bar, or play the video game machine in the corner.

No, I spent my money on something typically kept behind the convenience store's counter.

Playboy magazine, mostly. Sometimes Penthouse. And occasionally Hustler, though for some reason the clerk was sometimes unwilling to sell me that one.

Most men still remember their first wet dream. I remember mine vividly.

I remember it scared the hell out of me. Back then there was no such thing as sex education in the schools. At least not in my small town smack in the middle of the Bible belt.

I don't remember the dream specifically, as in who was in it, but I remember it woke me up in the middle of the night. It felt amazing, yet left this huge... mess, for lack of a better word.

I was convinced there was something wrong with me, and for days I wondered whether I should go see a doctor, yet was too afraid to explain what had happened to my parents.

A couple of weeks later, in an effort to recreate the incredible feeling I had at the end of my wet dream, I masturbated for the very first time.

While looking intently at the body of Miss July.

That started a sexual journey for me. From that moment on, until about two years ago, I had sex on a regular basis. Usually with a partner, but with myself when I was between partners or when it was just more expedient that way.

Looking back, I honestly can't remember not ejaculating at least once a week since that day.

I wasn't addicted to sex. Not in my opinion, anyway.

I just enjoyed the feeling I got when I got an erection. I enjoyed it even more when I felt a woman's touch on it. And even more yet when that woman took me into her mouth or vagina. For those two things, in my mind, were as much a surrender as anything else a woman could do.

It was a way of her saying, without necessarily verbalizing so, that she accepted me. She cared about me. She wanted to share with me things she shared with few others.

It made me feel special.

Only once in my younger years do I ever remember being unable to get an erection.

I was about twenty or so. It was a couple of years before I met Michelle and fell in love with her.

On this particular night I was on a date with a woman named Peggy. She was willing. I wasn't, because I was in the throes of a major flu.

To make it worse, my testicles were empty. I'd emptied them myself a day or two before. Between my masturbating shortly before my date and my feeling miserable, it just wasn't happening.

Peggy wanted intercourse, but it obviously wasn't going to happen. She tried oral, but didn't have much luck with that either.

She was nice about it, but I could see... something on her face. Not quite disgust, maybe. But more a feeling I'd let her down. She was disappointed, and I'd left her unsatisfied. I gave her oral sex and was able to make her climax (twice, as I remember), But still, I left her wanting.

I saw her later and we talked about it. I apologized, for the hundredth time, and told her I'd like to have another chance. But she was dating another man at that time, so a second chance just wasn't in the cards.

It so happened we shared a psychology class together. That's how we met.

As psychology majors, we knew the importance of talking things out, and we had a frank discussion.

I felt somewhat inadequate that night, despite my suspicions it was mostly brought on by circumstance.

She, on the other hand, felt she wasn't up to the task. That she wasn't capable enough. Or wasn't sexy enough. Or just didn't know how to turn me on.

And therein lies the rub.

A major part of the problem of ED isn't that it lessens our ability to feel good; to do the things we enjoy. That's part of it, sure.

But a major part of the problem, and I contend the biggest part of the problem, isn't the nice way it doesn't let us feel. It's the rotten way it makes us feel.

Let's face it.

The guilt is what gets us. The feelings of inadequacy. The feeling we've let down a loved one.

That is why ED sucks.

Peggy and I remained friends, although I lost track of her many years ago. For a long time I regretted not having that second chance with her to prove to her I wasn't a loser.

And I never forgot that day or how it made me feel.

I'm fifty eight now, and that day is long in my past. The very fact I can remember it so vividly is testament to a couple of things. First, it affirms the feelings of guilt and inadequacy we as men feel whenever we're unable to perform.

And second, it reflects the importance of sex throughout my adult life. Not only the act of sex itself, but also of my desire to please my lover.

My lover, for many years now, has been Michelle. We married after only a few weeks of meeting. We fell that much in love. And my love for Michelle has never faltered, never waivered. I've never cheated on her, and never will. She is my partner, my lover, my everything.

Just as we matched instantly as life partners, we also came together (no pun intended) quite well as lovers. It was an easy transition for us. We found we enjoyed the same things, shared the same passions, and both had an exceedingly strong desire to please the other.

In the beginning, we, to coin a common phrase, "went at it like rabbits." It was immensely enjoyable those first couple of years.

After that, the newness wore off and we slowed down a bit.

That wasn't to say the passion wasn't there. It was rather, I think, we came to realize that neither of us was going anywhere. That we didn't have to attack sex with the wild abandonment one might if it were in danger of going away.

We stopped trying, as another common phrase goes, to "wear that sucker out."

We settled into a habit of making love two to three times a week, when one or the other of us was in the mood and initiated it.

It was always, without fail, fulfilling and pleasurable.

Then came the summer of 2012. I began a book signing tour of Western Europe, followed immediately by a lecture tour across Great Britain.

The two combined kept me far from home for a total of nine months.

Michelle, because she was caring for her sick father and because of other career commitments back home, was unable to join me.

Except for seven very passionate days in Paris early into my book tour that I'll always cherish as one of my best memories.

The point is we were apart for several months. I could have strayed, as many in my position might have. But I'd never cheated on Michelle before, and never will.

In my younger (and even middle aged years) I was quite adept at masturbating, but those days were largely gone.

The result was that in the summer of 2012, and the winter and spring of 2013, I stopped getting erections.

And that was okay, for I had no need of them at the time.

Looking back, though, it might have been a very serious mistake.

For it was at the end of my trip to Europe, after I flew back to the States from London, that my erectile dysfunction began.

Looking back, I realize now that my inactivity might have played a key role in my ability to get a "hard-on."

If I had a chance to go back and do things differently, I still wouldn't have cheated on my wife. Faithfulness has been one of the basic cornerstones of our relationship from the beginning.

No, I wouldn't have strayed.

But I definitely would have revived my old habit of pleasuring myself.

I didn't. And I feel I paid a heavy price for it.

I've discussed this with many of my colleagues and friends. A lot of them maintain that the timing of the two things- my extended trip to Europe and onset of my ED- to be merely coincidence.

Perhaps they're right.

But I don't think so. I don't believe in coincidences.

I returned to the States on May 15th, 2013, completely unable to obtain an erection. That night was supposed to be my big homecoming. I was to wine and dine Michelle and then make love to her until the sun came up.

I did make love to her that night. I was able to pleasure her in many different ways. But none- not a single one- involved my penis. It, unfortunately, was deader than a doornail.

Another factor which may or may not have played a role in my ED is my diabetes.

I missed my annual physical in 2012. I normally do it in August of each year, and I was signing books in Germany at the time.

I didn't think too much of it. I felt as good as any other man I knew of my age.

Instead of having a physical done upon my return from Europe, I simply waited until August 2013.

It was at that physical I learned I had Type 2 diabetes.

It wasn't the end of the world. I was told I could probably avoid taking medication as long as I controlled my diet and changed some bad eating habits (Farewell, Snickers bars).

That my erectile dysfunction reared its very ugly head just a couple of months before made me wonder whether they were linked.

They say that everything is timing, and the timing of those three things (my extended abstinence, my ED and my diabetes) has made me wonder... what caused what else to happen?

Did the abstinence cause my inability to get an erection? Or was it the diabetes? Or was it a combination of both?

We've all heard the old saying, "Use it or lose it."

It's widely believed that the saying pertains directly to the male penis. And that it warns men against taking a long hiatus for sex. For such a long hiatus tells the body, essentially, that it no longer has need of a hard-on.

And that, sadly, the body responds as one would expect it to.

By saying, "Okay. If you don't need it any more we'll just take that ability away from you."

And it's pretty darn hard to get the cats back into the bag once they've been let out.

It's just as possible in my case that my ED wasn't caused by my abstaining at all. That it was caused by the onset of my diabetes.

Erectile dysfunction is, after all, one of the symptoms of diabetes.

It was a double whammy if there ever was one.

Michelle told me, "It's okay, honey. It's just something that happens when men get older. We can survive without it."

But I didn't want to survive without it. Sex had always been a very enjoyable part of our relationship, and it wasn't something I wanted to say goodbye to.

I told her so and she said, "Well, let's do everything we can do to fight it then."

That's the tact we took when we declared war on my ED.

We won that war, and are back to enjoying a very fulfilling sex life two or three times a week.

It was well worth the fight.

From Michelle:

I vividly remember the night he came home from London. I would have preferred he come back early in the day, so we could have a nice relaxing dinner and cocktails before a "welcome home" romp in the bedroom.

But because of the time difference he didn't land in New York City until 10:30 p.m.

I could have waited in Atlanta for him, but he would have had a layover and had to take a morning flight into Hartsfield the next day.

I didn't want to wait that long to see him, and we hadn't visited the Big Apple in awhile. So I chose to fly to New York to greet him.

I booked a nice mid-town hotel for a week and the plan was to play tourist, see some shows, see the Statue of Liberty (because despite half a dozen previous visits, I still had never been there).

And to spend a considerable amount of time in bed.

On the night of his arrival, by the time we claimed his bags and got back to the hotel it was past midnight.

By unspoken agreement, we decided to forego the physical romance and enjoyed a drink (actually a couple) on our balcony. He was too wound up from the travel to sleep, and I was too excited to sleep, so we looked out on the New York skyline and talked well into the night.

As I recall, we slept into the early afternoon the next day and would have slept longer had our hungry stomachs not awakened us.

We saw a play off Broadway that evening (not a very good one), had a pleasant dinner and retired to our room to have some fun.

The thing I remember most about that night, and the entire trip to New York, really, was my overwhelming feeling of guilt.

It never, not even once, occurred to me that perhaps there was a medical reason for his failure to get hard. Or maybe his fatigue from the long flight. Or maybe the fact he hadn't used it in awhile.

All I knew, in every fiber of my being, was that for the first time I could remember I failed him. I couldn't get him hard.

I hope I don't offend anyone with my language here. If I do, I'll apologize in advance. I grew up calling it a dick or a cock. It's natural for me, therefore, to continue to call it such. I've always considered the term penis so... clinical.

And after all, we're all adults here and this is a very adult discussion we're having. We might as well talk as most adults do.

I remember that night, holding his dick in my hand.

We were in our fifties, and I knew it wouldn't spring to life as it did when we were younger (I used to love it when we were in our twenties and he was rock-hard all the time). But still, the night before he left for Europe it had taken only a few seconds for him to begin to rise.

I had no reason to believe that on this night things would be any different.

It was flaccid, as it sometimes was, when we began our foreplay. That wasn't a problem, as I considered myself an expert at stimulating him. I remember I wore a new nightgown that night. It was short, and sheer. Not quite the lingerie you see on prominent display at those upscale mall stores (you know which ones I'm talking about), but considerably sexier than what Jacob was used to seeing me wear.

He told me I was beautiful and lifted my hair to kiss the scruff of my neck.

Those four things together... his kissing my neck, his eliciting my moan, my attire, and my gently massaging his cock, should have been enough to make him rock hard.

Any two of those things would have done the trick before he left for his extended trip.

But on this particular night it just wasn't happening.

His dick just wasn't playing ball.

We didn't let it stop us from doing other things, of course. He gave me oral sex for a considerable time and left me breathless. Yet even as I was in the throes of orgasm I remember feeling guilty that he was unable to find the same degree of pleasure.

I went down on him as well that night. His dick, though flaccid, still tasted the same. I love the way he tastes- always have. And to my knowledge my sucking him had never failed to give him an erection in the past.

On this night, though, it was a failure.

Oh, it stirred a couple of times. It even grew just a bit, although it never got hard enough for penetration.

And penetration was what we wanted the most that night.

We'd always, since the early days of our relationship, considered intercourse the best part of our lovemaking. It was the entree in our four course meal. The star on top of our Christmas tree. The thing which made us look forward to going to bed at night and which made us smile the next day.

Jacob always said we were as well suited sexually as any couple could be. I always loved the way he felt inside me and almost felt deprived when he had to leave me. He was talented, in that way... slow and gentle when I wanted him to be, yet capable of a ferocity which quite literally rocked my world (and left dents in the bedroom wall from the bed frame banging against it).

He was a patient lover as well. Although he knew that sometimes it was difficult for me to have an orgasm during intercourse, he always held himself back until I had done so at least once. Usually twice. And when he was ready he timed his so we could climax together: in my mind, the most joyful way to finish a night of lovemaking.

This particular night wasn't so joyous. My oral stimulation wasn't helping, and it finally dawned on me that the reason he was trying to draw away wasn't because it didn't feel good to him.

But rather it was embarrassing to him.

One of the things he told me later was that there was nothing sexy about my sucking a limp dick. And that he asked me to stop because he assumed it wasn't enjoyable to me.

I assured him that wasn't the case. I told him that I loved the way he tasted. And that he tasted the same whether he was hard or flaccid.

But he had this look on his face. He was humiliated and perhaps a little bit depressed.

It was a look I'd never seen before that night, but would see many more times in the coming months.

He kept apologizing. He kept saying he didn't know what was happening. Perhaps it was the time change. Or maybe the alcohol. He didn't drink much in Europe because he'd always hated drinking alone. And we had several cocktails that evening before we started our foreplay. So perhaps that was it, he said.

I, on the other hand, was apologizing as well.

I felt as though perhaps I wasn't sexy enough. Wasn't pretty enough. I remember actually getting out of bed at one point and going to the bathroom, where I stood before the mirror and examined my face.

Had I gotten that much older during he months he was gone? Had I gotten so much uglier that he no longer found me attractive?

I examined every wrinkle, every gray hair, trying to remember what I'd looked like months before, before he left.

It occurred to me that I was a hideous old hag. Of course he didn't find me attractive. Why would he?

I felt I must have aged a dozen years in those few short months.

I returned to the bed feeling defeated. I'd let him down. I wanted so much for his homecoming to be special. To be perfect. To be filled with warm memories we'd talk about many years into the future.

Instead, I let him down.

It was all my fault.

The last thing I remember about that night was falling asleep on his chest, his dick cupped in my hand. I assumed that at some point it would spring to life, waking both of us up so we could try again.

When I woke up the next morning he was already up, sitting on the balcony and drinking his morning coffee.

He was deep in thought.

I never was much good at reading minds, but I was pretty sure I knew the things going through his mind that particular morning.

He felt like a failure. And so did I.

For the next few days his flaccid dick became the key topic of discussion. We sat on a bench in Central Park and worried together whether it was just a temporary condition or might be permanent.

On a crowded ferry I very subtly rubbed my body against his, hoping I could stimulate him. I felt the bulge in his pants but it never got any larger.

My first trip to the Statue of Liberty was ruined, largely to disappointment and my own feelings of inadequacy.

The last night we were in New York City we had dinner plans, then cancelled them at the last minute. We were in our room, searching site after site on the internet, trying to find the answers to our questions and to see if there was any validity to our concerns.

And we had lots of concerns. It wasn't just the fact that intercourse had always been very enjoyable for both of us, and not something either of us wanted to give up.

No, there was much more to it than that.

He felt like a failure, that he could no longer perform for me. This was despite my reassurances that he could still please me sexually in so many other ways.

I, on the other hand, felt totally inadequate. I felt I was no longer attractive to him. No longer sexy. My memory went back to the days when I'd bathe in the tub, and he'd walk into the bathroom to shave. He'd see my naked body in the mirror as he shaved, and I'd watch his dick as he did so. I was always fascinated by his dick, both because I found it extremely sexy and because I was intrigued by the way the whole thing worked.

Anyway, in those days all it took was his seeing my wet and naked body in the tub to get his flaccid dick erect. Usually within seconds, with no touching, no stimulation of any kind.

I couldn't help remembering that and comparing it with our new situation. My fondling it didn't help. My sucking it helped a little, but not much.

I understood his feelings of failure, for I felt the same.

I felt ugly. And old. And worthless.

I was so bothered, those first few weeks, that my mind ran away with me. I became irrational.

I became jealous for the very first time in my life.

I knew, in my heart and my soul, that Jacob had always been completely devoted and faithful to me.

He'd never strayed, not even once, in all the time we'd been together.

But then again, I'd never given him a reason to stray.

And now, in my panicked mind, he had one.

For weeks I let my imagination run away from me. I had dreams of him looking for someone younger, someone sexier, someone capable of making his cock rock hard simply by his looking at her naked body.

I began to wonder whether it was possible everything we had was gone.

Whether he might be out there looking for my replacement.

So he could trade me in, like a used car with too many miles on it.

We sat down one night and I voiced my concerns. He took me in his arms and kissed me. First tenderly, then with passion. We made love, and it was wonderful. But there was no intercourse, and that diminished the joy. It felt good physically, but neither of us could deny there was a major piece of it that was missing.

It turned out we each blamed ourselves.

For something that was the fault of neither one of us.

That was the night we decided that we enjoyed the sensation of him being inside me too much to just give up on it.

We didn't know what we were up against. Had no clue, really, what it was or what it would take to defeat it.

But we decided to fight it anyway.

Chapter 1:   What is ED, Anyway?

And why does it think it has the right to swoop in and suck the joy out of our marriage?

In clinical terms, Erectile Dysfunction doesn't sound like the hideous monster it really is.

The American Medical Association describes it as such:

Erectile dysfunction or impotence is sexual dysfunction characterized by the inability to develop or maintain an erection of the penis during sexual activity in humans. A penile erection is the hydraulic effect of blood entering and being retained in sponge-like bodies within the penis. The process is most often initiated as a result of sexual arousal, when signals are transmitted from the brain to nerves in the penis. The most important organic causes are cardiovascular disease and diabetes, neurological problems (for example, trauma from prostatectomy surgery), hormonal insufficiencies (hypogonadism) and drug side effects.

Medical speak. Yucko.

But let's break the definition down for some clues how to treat the problem.

Ask a dozen people what the most powerful part of the human body is and you'll get a slew of different answers.

Many will say the human heart. After all, it works twenty four hours a day for every day of your life without ever taking a day off or even an hour to rest. Pretty powerful indeed.

Many will say the lungs, and for the very same reasons. The lungs never stop, unless we intentionally try to stop breathing by holding our breath. And all that does is make us pass out, at which times the lungs will start us breathing again without our permission. Ask any kid throwing a tantrum whether it's possible to hold their breath until they die. It isn't. The lungs are our friends and allies. And pretty powerful ones at that.

Body builders and those into physical fitness may say the legs are the most powerful parts of our human bodies. And that may be true, if you're talking about sheer brute strength. The upper legs contain our most powerful muscle groups. Try doing a dead lift without the aid of the legs. Most people on a leg machine can leg press more than their body weight. The legs are powerful indeed.

But only those who say the brain, or more specifically the human mind, pass this particular quiz.

The human brain weighs little more than a cheeseburger, yet determines whether we live or die. It drives every decision we make. It powers everything our body does, whether consciously or subconsciously. Think about it. It keeps our body functioning even when we sleep. It is the control center of us. Without our brain we're nothing but a big slab of meat.

Want to know how powerful the human brain is?

You can actually will yourself to death.

Don't believe me? Consider all of those people who've been in relatively good health, until they meet a major goal or milestone.

How many times have you read about the lady in the local newspaper who was ninety five years old?

And who tells the reporter she wants to make it to a hundred? And she lives another five years, and then passes away quietly in her sleep a few days after her hundredth birthday party?

Or the couple who's been married sixty years, then passes away within days of each other.

In the first case, the old lady had a goal she was determined to reach before she died. Once it was reached, she was content. She'd won. She'd conquered her goal. There was no longer any more reason to fight off the inevitable.

In the latter case, the first half of the couple finally succumbed to old age. The second half merely gave up, not wanting to go on without him or her. And simply willed himself or herself into eternal sleep.

The AMA says that erectile dysfunction is *"is most often initiated as a result of sexual arousal, when signals are transmitted from the brain to nerves in the penis."*

So, then, the brain is where the erection starts. Not the penis, as most would believe.

The brain is the boss in this and every other case. The mind is our enemy or our friend when it comes to ED. We can give up and accept ED as inevitable. Or we can use our mind as our friend and ally. We can decide we will not suffer the disappointment and humiliation of a flaccid penis. And we will find ways to work with the mind (and sometimes trick it) into achieving our goal.

Let's focus now on working with it.

We work with our mind by opening it up. Opening it up to explore new techniques and methods which have been known to aid in our impotence problem.

And then to go one step further to try new things. Things we may have never thought of before.

Only when you consider all the possible courses of action as tools to help you with the problem can you find the right combination of tools to fix the problem.

You don't go to fix your broken car armed only with a screwdriver.

You take a tool box full of tools, because you don't know what you might encounter or what you might need.

Fixing erectile dysfunction applies the same principle.

Fill up your toolbox with a variety of tools. Then figure out which ones you need, and get them working together.

Every one of us is different. What works on one of us may or may not work on another.

The trick is to gather as many tools as possible, then to find which ones work on your particular body. In all likelihood, it'll take several such tools, working in tandem, to get your penis functioning again.

We found our set of tools. Now we're going to help you find yours.

But you have to keep an open mind. You have to be willing to consider everything.

If you're not willing to do that, you've already given up.

Chapter 2:   Back to that whole "Keep an open mind" thing:

Here's a prime example.

Once we decided we were going to declare our own personal war on erectile dysfunction we saw our first step as finding out all we could about the various techniques for treating it.

We made a pact going in... no matter how outlandish or bizarre the treatment was, we'd at least consider it rationally before we cast it out.

We looked to see whether it had merit. Meaning, did it come from a reasonably reliable source. Was it written up in any medical journals? Was it the result of a study somewhere? And if so, where was the study performed? Was it conducted, for example, at a known college or university? Or was it studied by a manufacturer trying to push its own product?

We looked to see what the claimed results were. And whether the results were believable. We tried to shy away from outlandish claims, such as magical pills which promised to, in their words, "make your dick hard as a rock, and make it four inches longer too." Size wasn't our problem. Getting and keeping an erection was.

We looked not only at American and British methods and techniques and products, but those all over the world. Our thinking was that people in the U.S. or England don't have a monopoly on ED, although we do seem to have way more than our share of pricks (most of them in political office or the recording industry). Some of the best techniques, believe it or not, came from the Asian countries. They seem to take ED very seriously over there. Perhaps that explains why China has so many people.

We looked at oral stimulants and supplements with a wary eye. We were open to any and all suggestions, but didn't want to put anything in Jacob's mouth which might be harmful to him.

Those were our guidelines as we pored over medical journals, dove head first into the internet, and queried both of our doctors, as well as several personal friends in the medical field.

One of our discoveries (and one of our favorites), applies a very common-sense approach.

It reminds us that the penis is, in essence, a muscle. In that respect, it's not much different than our arms and legs.

Well, there is some difference. We don't try to stuff an arm or a leg into a vagina. That would be painful.

If we don't exercise our legs, for example, they become soft and lazy. If we don't exercise them for a long enough period of time, they begin to atrophy.

Eventually, they become useless.

The Japanese applied the same logic to the penis. The longer we don't use it, the lazier and less cooperative it becomes. If we exercise it by using it frequently, it can react (sometimes, not always) in the same manner those legs will if we start walking or working them out at the gym.

In other words, it may be possible your penis is just out of shape from disuse or too-infrequent use.

So what to do?

According to the Japanese, we need to get it erect or semi-erect, even if it's just temporary and we don't do anything with it.

And we need to do it several times a day.

That's why this was one of our most favorite techniques.

We called this our "Ed Project." As in Ed, the name, not the condition. It became an innocuous way of referring to a thing that had important implications, while at the same time was rather fun. It became somewhat of a game for us.

From Michelle:

I've always loved playing with Jacob's dick. I think part of it was penis envy, as cliché as that may sound. It always kind of pissed me off a bit that I didn't have one of my very own. I was jealous of guys because they had one and I didn't.

The other part of it was... well, I just liked playing with it. It gave him pleasure. It made me wet. It led to lovemaking before the ED monster came into our lives. And it became my best hope of getting Jacob's dick back on track.

Our goal was to make him hard or semi-hard eight to ten times a day. It didn't matter how or where, or how long he stayed hard. But rather just to get him there.

It wasn't much different than going to the gym and working your arms or your legs.

Except that if you worked your dick at the gym you'd likely cause quite a stir.

Usually I have the first turn of each day, because I almost always wake up first.

I find his dick under the covers and begin fondling it. It almost always starts to stir immediately. I remember to caress his balls also, because that helps him to get hard as well.

I stimulate his dick in a variety of ways, since what works great one day might not work at all the next.

If I need to I'll crawl under the covers and suck him, or climb on top of him and rub his dick against my clit.

Some of that (or all of it) always works to get him at least semi-hard.

Then, to use a rather harsh sounding term, I drop him like a hot potato.

It's not to be mean.

It's to get him back into the habit of getting hard. And by doing it several times a day it becomes more of a habit, and helps get this particular muscle (my favorite one) back into shape.

From Jacob:

As I said earlier, I masturbated a lot as a teenager. I think we all did. At least all of us guys. Most men would be embarrassed to admit that, but I believe it to be true.

I'd gotten (mostly) out of the habit of masturbating over the years, thanks mainly to finding Michelle and the great sex life we've enjoyed.

Over the past few years I've used masturbation mainly as an occasional tool. Say, for example, when I was in the mood but Michelle was sound asleep and I didn't want to wake her. Or when I was in the mood and she was sick or out of town on a business trip.

My penis and my right hand were no longer the frequent partners they once were. They became more like friends with benefits.

One of the primary reasons I blame myself for my ED was because I should have seen it coming and prevented it. I firmly believe in the "use it or lose it" principle. I should have masturbated frequently when I was abroad. I didn't. I didn't use it, therefore I lost it.

Maybe. We'll never really know. But whether that was the main cause or not, I did indeed lose it.

And I was determined to get it back.

So I was as excited as Michelle about the theory that by exercising the penis several times a day, we might be able to "get it back into shape."

As Michelle said, she typically fondles me first thing in the morning. I have to say, even after all these years it's the best way to wake up. Far better than coffee, even.

Sometimes her morning fondling leads to sex, since I've gotten my hard-ons back. As often than not, though, it's just a pleasant way to wake up.

On the days when we make love, I typically ejaculate and then he's down for the count for the rest of the day.

On the days when we don't enjoy a great round of early morning sex, she fondles me until I'm erect and then abandons me.

That may sound harsh, but that's the technique. And it, when combined with other things, seems to work.

That's not the end of it. According to the Japanese study it must be done at least six times a day. Eight to ten is the optimal amount.

I typically make myself hard again in my morning shower, using the "massage" option on my shower head to help with the process. I don't allow myself to ejaculate, though, stopping just short of it.

At least twice a day, while I'm at work, I lock my office door and turn on some internet porn to help stimulate me, then fondle myself to erection. Then, just when it really starts being fun, I stop.

I'm a prick tease.

This continues when we get home from work. If it's my turn to cook dinner, Michelle will sometimes come up behind me and reach around to play with my penis. This is facilitated, of course, by the fact that I've taken up the habit of running around the house nude on the nights we're not expecting company.

More on that later.

If Michelle is cooking I typically masturbate (but not to completion. Never to completion) while she's doing so.

After dinner, if we're not going out, we generally watch TV to catch up on the news, and sometimes stream one of our favorite shows to watch.

One of the many nice things about being married to Michelle is that she never seems to tire of having her hands on my body.

She says it's one of her favorite things.

It's one of mine too.

While we're watching TV she gently kneads my testicles or plays with my penis in a variety of ways. Sometimes she goes down on me. Sometimes she merely rests her hand upon it.

Sometimes she pauses when it becomes hard, and that's okay.

Sometimes she takes me farther, and relies on me to tell her when I'm getting close so she'll know when to back off.

According to the theory, this method not only helps the penis to "relearn" the act of getting erect. It also helps stimulate the testicles. Which, in turn, makes them produce semen. Which, in turn, increases the pressure in the testicles, since they'll want to eject the semen and get rid of it.

Having your testicles full or partially full of semen helps stimulate the penis, since they work closely together.

And that, of course, helps the whole process.

So, then, to recap...

One technique we used successfully on the long journey to my (our) recovery was the technique of frequent penis stimulation. At least six times a day is recommended, with eight to ten times per day being the optimal goal.

For us, this was one of the most fun techniques in our ED Tool Box, because it required seemingly constant physical touching, which we both (as it turns out) love.

As an added benefit, it was something we could do together. Versus, for example, me taking a pill and hoping for the best.

To that regard, it enabled us to put forth a united front... teamwork, if you will... and gave us a sense we were working together to help defeat the ED monster.

Erectile Dysfunction Tool Box Thus Far: 1 Item

1. Frequent penis stimulation

Chapter 3:   *Continuing* with that whole "Keep an open mind" thing:

A little pain can go a long way.

Men are like snowflakes.

No two are alike.

And just as men have their own preferences when it comes to, say, the foods they like to eat, the same can be said for their sexual appetites.

Some men, when it comes to choosing a sexual partner, prefer blondes (reminds us of an old movie…). Some men prefer brunettes or redheads.

For some men, they don't care. They're desperate and just want to get laid, and don't much care what their partner looks like.

Most men, while they may have a preference in hair color, wisely use several other factors when choosing a partner. Whether the chemistry is there. Whether there's something other than sex on which to base a relationship. Whether there's the promise for love. Whether the partner is stable and caring and a good person.

The same preferences hold true for short partners or tall ones. Caucasian, black or Asian partners. Thin or a few extra pounds.

Every man is different. Every woman is different.

We select our sexual partners, and our life partners as well, based on those preferences.

And just for the record, there's nothing wrong with having preferences. After all, preferences are nothing more than a process with which we can "weed out" the noncompatible.

Let's take that one step further.

Just as men have their preferences for sexual partners, they also have their personal preferences for the type of sex they like to have.

Most men want their penis gently massaged. Or tenderly kissed. They love to feel their manhood kneaded, a tongue or soft lips upon the head. That same tongue and same soft lips working their way up and down his shaft.

But not all men are that way.

Some men are a little more daring. A bit more reckless.

In the same way some men put hot sauce on their food and others don't, some men like a bit of excitement (for lack of a better term) in their sexual repertoire.

The Chinese have been toying with the idea of using acupuncture needles to gently poke the head of a penis to stimulate it. It's not for everyone, but for a surprising number, it works very well.

From Michelle:

I was with several men before Jacob came along. With most of them it was nothing serious. I was engaged to one man, though, two years before I met Jacob. I realized he wasn't the man I thought he was, and I broke off the engagement. He wound up going to prison for crimes of anger and was there for several years. I've thanked God many times over the years for getting out of that relationship for a couple of reasons.

First of all, had I not broken up with the man I might well have been the target of some of that anger.

And secondly, I never would have had the chance to meet and fall madly in love with Jacob, who is and always will be the man of my dreams.

I only mention my past relationships as a precursor to this: There were other men before Jacob. Jacob did not take my virginity and was far from my first.

But Jacob's dick is the only one which ever scared me.

The first time I saw it I thought I'd never be able to accommodate it. I did, of course, but that first time had me worried.

One of the things we realized early on was that his size (and the fact I have a very small mouth) was going to be an issue. Try as I might, I couldn't avoid my teeth getting in the way. I occasionally bit him or scraped my teeth against him.

I certainly didn't mean to, at least not at first. It just happened.

When it did I apologized, and worried that I hurt him. He finally told me he rather liked it. It didn't hurt him at all, and that it added a little bit of "spice" (as he called it) to an otherwise ordinary blow job.

Mind you, I never bit him hard enough to draw blood or to cause him any serious or permanent damage.

But he did enjoy it. So when I stumbled across a Chinese method of using pins to stimulate a flaccid penis into having an erection, I thought this might be something he'd be willing to try.

From Jacob:

You have to remember it was the Chinese who invented acupuncture, which is used to relieve pain all over the world. I myself have never tried acupuncture, and would probably be the last one to subscribe to it.

But I don't have an aversion to pain, in limited intensity and limited doses, as a part of a normal and healthy sexual diet.

Michelle mentioned her tendency to accidentally bite me or to scrape me with her teeth while having sex.

She was quite surprised when I told her I enjoyed it. Now then, I never told her to intentionally chew on the darned thing. But an occasionally nip was quite pleasurable to me.

I told her I equated it with my dietary tastes. Some men don't like spicy foods. I, on the other hand, love them. I pour hot sauce on my hot sauce, and still complain that my food is bland.

Perhaps I like my sex the same way.

A tiny stab of pain is served best when you don't know it's coming. That leads me to believe that the buildup, or anticipation, is what makes the act itself more pleasurable.

Apparently the technique was developed not by acupuncturists or medical professionals, but by university students experimenting with their own ideas for might bring life back to a flaccid penis.

Michelle suggested we try it, and I, being the open-minded kind of guy I am, readily agreed.

The technique involves manual stimulation, punctuated occasionally (several times per minute) with a gentle poke from the tip of a pin to the head of the penis. Always in a different place, so that the owner of the penis doesn't know when the next stick is coming, or where.

Just as I think the anticipation of a nip from my wife during oral sex adds to the pleasure, I believe the mysterious nature of this technique adds to the stimulation.

I might note that we didn't run out and buy a set of acupuncture needles. We didn't want to purchase something we'd never use again if we didn't like the technique or it didn't work for us.

Instead, Michelle visited the sewing and notions aisle at our local Walmart and bought a container of little stick pins with colorful ball heads, about an inch or so long.

She started by massaging my penis as I lay back on the bed with my eyes closed. In one hand she held my penis and in the other hand the pin, so she was able to poke me when and where the mood struck her.

I have to say, this was one of the most enjoyable of all the techniques we tried.

I'll be the first to recognize this might not be for everybody, but I thoroughly enjoyed it, and it definitely worked for me. Only one time did it fail to make me semi-erect (or better), and that was just two days after we had sex and I ejaculated completely. That was before I learned the technique of holding some back, which we'll talk about later. My testicles were more or less empty, which doesn't bode well for any efforts to obtain an erection.

I should also point out that this isn't the massive stab of agonizing pain that many of you may imagine it to be.

There is no blood. The pin never breaks the skin nor leaves any marks.

I would equate the actual pain it generates to feeling not unlike the bite of a mosquito.

Except in this case, you get to keep your blood.

Remember, keeping an open mind is key to finding what works for you. Discard this idea if you wish. But as I said, it's one of the things which worked best for me.

And who knows? You just might decide you like it.

Erectile Dysfunction Tool Box Thus Far: 2 Items

1. Frequent penis stimulation
2. Pin stimulation to penis head

Chapter 4:   *Develop an ongoing dialog with your doctor.*

He can be your penis's best friend.

I've known my primary care physician for over fifteen years. I consider him a good friend, and frequently see him socially in addition to in the exam room.

He's a good man, and I trust him, quite literally, with my life.

Here's why: he's fond of telling our mutual friends that he wants me to live forever. Because I'm the only person on earth he can beat (occasionally) on the golf course.

Having a healthy relationship and a rapport with your doctor can help you tremendously when it comes to beating the ED monster. Because if you're comfortable with him, you're more likely to ask the types of embarrassing questions you should be asking.

If he considers you a friend, or at least a cut above the cattle who file through his office disguised as patients day in and day out, he's more likely to provide you better care.

Here's an interesting statistic: It's estimated that twenty four percent of men who have ED don't ever talk about it to their physicians. They choose to ignore it and hope it goes away (Here's a hint. It doesn't). Or, they consider it just a fact of life, a by-product of getting older.

And they never have it treated. They pretty much give up on their sex life and deprive themselves (and their spouse or significant other) of many joyful sexual adventures.

At that point, for those men, the ED monster becomes a lifelong curse.

On the other hand, talking to your doctor about it can benefit you in a myriad of ways.

And no, I'm not just talking about your inability to get Viagra or Cialis without his writing you a prescription.

That's a big part of it, yes. But he can also advise you on other methods that don't require prescription meds, and are perhaps better suited (and safer) for your particular medical needs.

From Jacob:

I remember the day I walked into Paul's office that morning. Paul isn't just my doctor. I also consider him a friend, and as such I feel comfortable talking to him about anything.

Our conversation went something like this:

Me: I haven't been performing well in the bedroom lately.

Him: Good. I've had my eye on Michelle for quite some time. Ask her if she's free on Friday night.

Me: I'm serious.

Him: Who says I'm not?

Me: And how is you fucking my wife going to fix my erection problem?

Him: It won't. But it'll make me very happy. And it'll make Michelle even happier. Maybe she'll make you an omelet or something to show you her appreciation.

Me: I think I need a new doctor.

Him: Okay. But I need Michelle's phone number before you go.

Paul and I have known each other for a long time. Granted, probably a lot longer than you've known your own doctor. Chances are you don't joke around like he and I do. But here's my point: He's a medical professional. He's used to fielding questions and providing good answers about all those embarrassing things you don't want to ask him.

But you HAVE to ask. He may know a lot of things about ED, or whatever else is ailing you. But one thing he's not good at is mindreading. If you don't tell him what the problem is, he can't help you fix it.

Most doctors would have prescribed ED medication and been done with it. They'd have said, "Here's a pill for you to take. Have fun. You'll get my bill. Goodbye."

Or, if you had medical issues that prevented you from getting the magical pill he'd have said, "Nothing I can do for you. You have a bad heart. Sorry, but you're out of luck. I'll send you a bill anyway. Goodbye."

Paul's not like that.

He asked me the specifics.

Him: How long has it been going on?

Me: It started a month ago, when I got back from London.

Him: How long were you abroad?

Me: For several months.

Him: Were you active while you were there?

Me: No. I'm faithful to Michelle.

Him: I know that, dummy. Were you spanking the monkey while you were there?

Me: Is that relevant?

Him: Very much so.

Me: No. I didn't think it was important.

Him: It probably would have helped. When you just dropped sex cold turkey, your body may have interpreted it as you deciding you weren't interested anymore.

Me: Is there any way I can get it back?

Him: Maybe. But we have to be careful because of your blockage and family history of heart disease. Also, you're a diabetic now. That's going to make it harder.

Me: Good. I want to make it harder.

Him: Not what I meant.

Me: I know… so what do we do?

Him: We start by doing the easy things. They sometimes help. Then we progress to the harder stuff.

Paul showed me that certain drugs can lead to ED, or make a minor ED problem worse.

Further, the way two drugs interact can do the same thing, although one or the other of the drugs, when prescribed alone, might not have any effect at all.

Lastly, he told ne that certain foods we eat can have an adverse affect on our ED problem.

Paul worked with me to show me how certain things we eat cause our bodies to do certain things.

For example, he told me that eating fatty foods clogs arteries. I already knew that, and was already cutting down on my fat intake because I have a partial blockage in one of my arteries.

But he told me eating the same fatty foods also causes people to sweat more.

I could relate. I'd noticed even before he mentioned it that I was sweating far less at the gym than I did before I started cutting back on fats.

He said sugar can do the same thing. It not only makes you fat and can lead to diabetes, it can also make you sweat profusely.

He said whenever he gets a complaint from a patient that they tend to sweat profusely, he prescribes a reduction in sugar and fatty foods and it solves the problem almost every time. Or at least reduces it to a great degree.

What does that have to do with our ED problem? Very little. But I mention it to show that the things we eat, without thinking, can have a major impact on our ED problem.

Like the aforementioned sugar.

Sugar is one of those things our body doesn't really need, but which we crave. (Caffeine is another). Paul says that's why our body sweats when we eat too much sugar. Sweating is one of the ways the body gets rid of the things it doesn't want or need.

The problem with sugar is that (in some men) it can prevent an erection. Or lessen the erection. And as we know, a penis that's only halfway erect might as well be not erect at all.

Paul advised me to get rid of all unnecessary sugar.

I do have a bit of a sweet tooth, so I asked him to define "unnecessary sugar."

He said that many foods have hidden sugars we don't even know are there. The example he used was ketchup.

I never knew ketchup was loaded with sugar, did you?

He said I'd never rid all sugar from my diet, because it's contained in so many of the things we consume without even knowing it.

But he said that getting rid of those things I eat specifically for the sugar, like candy bars and glazed donuts and ice cream, can help me in a myriad of ways.

First of all, since I'm diabetic now I shouldn't have them to begin with. I've known that for awhile, but have still been cheating occasionally. Who can say "no" to that Snicker's bar calling my name while I'm standing in line at the register?

So giving up sugar helps me to keep my blood sugar level in the 120 to 150 range he's having me shoot for.

Over the long term, giving up sugar will help me lose those extra twenty pounds Paul's been after me to lose for years.

And lastly, he says giving up sugar can help some men with their erection problem.

I don't know if I'm one of those men.

I just know that I cut back dramatically on my sugar intake, at the same time I did a lot of other things. My ED problem went away.

I'll never know for sure to what degree giving up sugar helped, because I was doing so many other things at the same time.

But here's the thing:

If you know that sugar is bad for you, and you know that getting rid of it (or most of it) can help you medically in so many ways, then why not give it up?

Reasons to eat sugar:
1. To satisfy a temporary craving that will soon go away on its own even if not satisfied

Reasons to give up sugar:
1. Reduces risk of diabetes
2. Reduces risk of heart disease
3. Reduces risk of damage to liver and kidneys
4. Helps to lose weight

5. Reduces excess sweating
6. May prevent or lessen severity of ED in men

Kind of a no brainer, isn't it?

Okay, let's put reduction of sugar intake on our list of things to do.

But there's so much more that Paul has done for me.

Paul is one of those doctors who doesn't believe in overtreatment. What I mean by that is, he doesn't just listen to your symptoms, make a calculated guess, issue you five different prescriptions, and then send you on your way.

Then follow you out the door so he can make his tee time.

Yes, there are doctors like that out there. Way too many of them.

Paul isn't one of them.

Paul thinks we (the world in general, but mostly Americans) are way overmedicated.

And he doesn't like prescribing medications unless they're absolutely necessary.

Seriously.

That's about his only redeeming quality, besides the fact he's lousy in poker.

Just kidding. The fact is, he's a great doctor. I hope he's ahead of his time, for I believe more doctors should do what Paul does and look for other means of treatment before he just prescribes potentially harmful meds willy nilly.

When I went to see him complaining of pain in my feet, he immediately suspected diabetic nerve pain. He sent me to the lab for a glucose test, and they made me drink some nasty orange stuff that made me want to vomit.

Sure enough, I had diabetes.

Most doctors would have said "Give up sugar" and prescribed some very harsh medicines, which would have treated the diabetes but had some potentially bad side effects. **Including ED.**

Paul did say "Give up sugar." But he also sent me to a dietician. He did give me a prescription, but it wasn't for medication. It was for a cool little machine about as big as my computer mouse, which I use to read my blood sugar each day. I didn't even know you could get a blood glucose meter with a prescription, but you can. My insurance even covered it, minus a six dollar co-pay.

The dietician taught me to eat better. And since I confessed to having a sweet tooth, she showed me ways to satisfy that sweet tooth without using sugar to do it.

For the foot pain he told me to go to a nutrition store and buy something called "Stabilized R-Lipoic Acid."

"There are several kinds and several brands," he said. "The brand doesn't matter. But be sure it has an R in front of the Lipoic Acid. That's the best one for you."

I didn't ask him what the "R" stood for or why that was important. I still don't know.

What I do know, though, is that I started taking the stuff (and wearing diabetic socks) and the foot pain went away within days. Bear in mind that before I saw Paul the pain was so severe it was keeping me up at night. I was popping half a dozen ibuprofen just to get to sleep.

Now it's gone completely.

And it's gone without any harsh prescription drugs which may help with one problem but cause others.

If you're on diabetic drugs, ask your doctor about R-Lipoic Acid. I recognize that we're all different, and that just because it worked well for me doesn't necessarily mean it'll work for you. But at least ask the question. You have nothing to lose. Except the possibility you'll be able to get off a harsh drug that's contributing to your ED...

Chapter 5: *If You Have a Family History of Heart Disease or Partial Blockage, Don't Skip This Chapter.*

It's Kind of Important.

While we're talking about Paul and some of the ways he treats his patients, we'll talk about heart disease and its affect on the penis.

Specifically, its ability to become erect and to stay that way.

The co-relation of the two isn't necessarily due to heart disease itself, although low blood pressure or partial blockage can reduce blood flow, and it's the blood inflow which makes your penis come alive.

Most of the reason men with heart issues or hypotension (low blood pressure) have problems with ED isn't the problem of low blood pressure itself.

Rather it's the side effects of the medication they take to treat the heart issues or hypotension.

Again, modern medicines are wonderful things. They save many lives each and every day. But nearly all of them have side effects. And in the case of men over fifty, an alarming number of those medicines list problems with impotency as one of those side effects.

Doctor Paul is a physician who doesn't believe in prescribing medications unless they're necessary. He tries other, less potentially harsh, methods first.

Your doctor should consider those methods as well.

We're not advocating you stop taking your prescribed meds.

What we're advocating is that you talk to your doctor. Tell him that you've been taking *Brand X* to treat your blood pressure problem. Tell him you checked the information pamphlet that the FDA requires be included in every new prescription, and that it lists impotency as a possible side effect. Tell him you've been suffering from ED and you want to know if there is another method of treatment that will protect your heart and still allow you to have sex.

He might say no. But in all likelihood he'll say, "You know what? We can try *Brand W*. It's less likely to contribute to your intimacy problems. Let's try it out for a while and see what happens."

A good doctor will listen to your concerns and try to work with you.

If he refuses to… if he says, "I prescribed that to you because it's the only thing that'll work for you," it might be time to seek a second opinion.

From Jacob:

Of course, the best option is no prescription medicines at all. But only your doctor can determine whether that's an option for you.

So far Paul has only prescribed one medication for me: Viagra, but he told me only to use it when everything else fails (which it occasionally does). It's our backup plan, which we use only every once in a while. Usually when I'm extra tired or we have sex two nights in a row.

More on that later.

Back to non-prescription alternatives to prescription medicines.

I'm fifty eight years old. And while I wish I was as healthy as I was in my twenties (and got erections several times a day even when I didn't want or need them), I'm like most men my age. I have a few medical problems. I mentioned the diabetes and the partial blockage, which Paul says we caught early enough to fix before it becomes a major problem. He also tells me my blood pressure is a bit higher than normal, and so is my cholesterol. He's closely monitoring those two things.

He's got me modifying my diet, which he says is the best thing I can do to help get healthier.

And the dietician he referred me to is the spitting image of Elizabeth Hurley, so I don't mind going to see her at all.

So I'm eating much better, which he assures me will help me live longer as well as helping with the ED problem.

And after all, that's precisely why I want to live longer. So I can solve the ED problem and have more sex with my lovely wife.

Hey, we all have our priorities...

Anyway, a diet heavy in veggies and fruits (more veggies than fruits if you're diabetic) and low in fats is a good thing. A very good thing.

Paul also had me get an over the counter supplement called Slo Niacin. It's good for the heart.

He's got me taking fish oil tablets for the same reason.

And he's got me exercising more.

I used to be a dedicated runner. For many years I ran a hundred miles a week or more.

I even ran in a marathon, in Honolulu, in 1981.

It damn near killed me, but I'm glad I did it.

These days I can't run. My knees are bad, no doubt a result of all those thousands of miles I ran in my youth.

But that's okay.

I can still walk, and Michelle and I walk around our neighborhood for a mile or so every evening.

And sometimes in the morning if we're awake and want to see the sunrise.

We also swim and ride bikes on nice days.

All of that is good for us.

At our age, we do what we can do, even if it's not what we once could.

All exercise is good exercise.

Bottom line: See your doctor. And don't be shy to tell him you're having erection problems.

He can't help you if he doesn't know.

From Michelle:

Men and women view the human body so much differently. We, as women, spend so much time being modest, wearing uncomfortable bras and panties, and constantly worrying that we'll reveal too much and be branded a shameless slut.

I once was horrified to learn part of my right nipple was exposed in a grocery store. I was so traumatized I wouldn't go shopping for weeks. And when I started going again I was paranoid for a long time. I looked at everyone I saw, wondering if they were there that day. Whether they saw my nipple. And whether they'd spread the word to all their friends that I was easy.

Men, on the other hand, don't care.

They'll whip that sucker out in a heartbeat, twirl it around a few times, then place bets with their friends on whose is bigger.

Don't believe me? Go on Facebook and see how many unsolicited penis pics you get from men you don't even know.

But here's what's really odd... as much as men like showing off and playing with and bragging about their dicks... they can be really shy when it comes to telling the doctor their little friend isn't working any more.

It's mind boggling, it really is. I mean, some of these guys' whole lives revolve around their penis and what they do with it.

Yet when it breaks they want to keep it under wraps.

Dumb, dumb, dumb.

Jacob says it's all related to pride, and the whole macho caveman thing. Men don't want to admit it when they can't perform, even when it means foregoing the help they need.

Sometimes they need a push from us, their significant others. After all, we miss that little sucker too.

Push him. Coerce him. Threaten him if you have to.

Mention that the produce guy at Ralph's winked at you the other day. The one who looks remarkably like George Clooney. And say that since you're no longer getting dick at home anyway...

Do whatever you have to do, or say whatever you have to say, to get your man to the doctor. And MAKE him talk about his ED problem when he gets there.

It's that important.

Erectile Dysfunction Tool Box Thus Far: 4 Items

1. Frequent penis stimulation
2. Pin stimulation to penis head
3. Eat well. Diet is everything
4. Enlist your doctor's help

Chapter 6:   *A Healthy Dose of Erotica at Bedtime Never Hurts.*

And it often helps...

Remember our agreement. Consider everything we discuss with an open mind. If you close your mind and discard something outright, you may be throwing away a possible solution to your ED problem without even considering it.

It's no different than when your kids refused to eat their broccoli at age six, remember?

You: Eat your broccoli.
Your kid: No.
You: Eat your broccoli, damn it.
Your kid: No.
You: Why not?
Your kid: I don't like it.
You: How do you know? You've never tried it.
Your kid: I just know I'm not gonna like it. It's green and lumpy and looks like a tree.
You: *If you never try new things, you'll never find new things that you love.*
Your kid tries it.
Your kid: Yum yum.

If you never try new things, you'll never find new things that you love...

From Michelle:

Jacob and I are authors by trade. We've been writing professionally for years. I started writing when I was a little girl and now I do it for a living. We have lots of friends who are authors as well. One of my best friends is Roxanna Holliman, who writes some of the best erotica available on Amazon.com.

I used to edit Roxanna's books for her, and Jacob would always ask to read her drafts when I was finished with them.

He always said he did so because he loved the story lines. He's into time travel and Albert Einstein and all that stuff so I kind of bought it at first.

But then I noticed that every time he sat in front of my computer and read through the drafts, he got a boner.

It turned out that erotica turned him on.

When he came back from his European tour (my words... it makes him sound like a rock star, doesn't it?) he had trouble getting an erection, and we decided to team up and do everything we could to combat the problem.

He's always said I have a very sexy voice, and we decided to experiment one night. He lay in bed and I read to him aloud a couple of chapters from "Times March," which was Roxanna's best seller at the time. While I read I fondled his cock.

Now, since he developed ED we've tried a variety of things. Usually my fondling doesn't, by itself, produce an erection. And to be truthful, fondling him while I read to him doesn't always work.

But it frequently does. The combination of physical pleasure and his closing his eyes and listening to my words excites him sometimes to get hard and stay that way for awhile.

I asked him why it works for him when my just rubbing his dick usually doesn't.

He said the rubbing is nice, but when he closes his eyes and listens to my words at the same time, he can picture himself in the scene with my characters, actually experiencing what they're experiencing as though he's one of the characters himself.

That was the basis for our looking for other erotica. He was able to find several other books which appealed to him as well.

He prefers books with a solid storyline. "Not just smut," he says. But something you'd enjoy reading even without the dirty parts.

This isn't something we do every night. But it is one of the many tools we have in what we call our "ED tool box."

Some nights we start our foreplay in this manner:

He'll lay face up upon the bed, his eyes closed and his body relaxed.

I'll lie next to him, but farther down on the bed, my face near his dick.

I'll massage his dick and his balls as I read, the book propped up on his stomach. Sometimes I'll take a break and suck on him a bit as well. He likes the occasional variation in my activities.

Sometimes if I'm reading a particular passage and feel him responding, I'll purposely go back a couple of pages and read the same passage again.

As I said, this sometimes works and it sometimes doesn't.

If his penis doesn't respond within, say, twenty minutes or so, we haven't really lost anything. After all, doing this particular thing is something we both enjoy tremendously even when it doesn't make his dick hard.

On the nights when he doesn't get an erection, we simply put the book aside and move onto another of our "tools."

And we keep going until we find one that works.

That brings up an important point.

Just as every man is different, every penis is different. They may all look more or less the same, but they respond to different stimuli.

And what makes our task as the partners who stimulate them even harder (no pun intended) is that what may work on a particular penis one night may not work at all the next night.

Cocks are wonderful. But as it turns out, they are terribly finicky.

That's why it's important to have a lot of tools at your disposal.

Try one thing. If it works, great. Enjoy a session of lovemaking and rejoice in it.

If it doesn't work, go on to something else. If you have enough tools, something will usually make your man hard. You just have to find the one thing, or combination of things, that's going to work on that particular night.

From Jacob:

Written erotica is a lot like porn. What stimulates one man might not stimulate another man at all. Also, a book which I find to be a turn-on on Tuesday may not appeal at all to me on Friday.

When I went shopping for erotica I looked for a variety of stuff. I wanted stories that were interesting enough to stand on their own even without the sex. I didn't want to be bored while Michelle was reading to me, and ruin the moment while falling asleep.

But at the same time, when she gets to the erotic parts of the book (What Michelle calls the "juicy parts") I wanted it to be descriptive enough to allow me to close my eyes and visualize her words.

At the same time, though, the written word is totally different than porn for one very distinctive reason.

When a man watches porn he frequently gets aroused, but it's hard to place himself into the picture.

In other words, when he watches a man make love to a beautiful woman on his television screen he can't visualize himself making love to her because the man is in the way.

But with erotica, when I close my eyes and listen to Michelle's words, the only two people in my mind are Michelle and I. There's no other man in the way. Her words, and her sexy voice, convince me that we're doing the things she says we're doing. Even if we've never done that particular act before. And her stimulating me with her hand heightens the effect.

Let me give you a quick example.

The scene she read me the other night had her two literary characters skinny dipping at a small lake. At night. In Paris, within view of the Eifel Tower.

It was part romance, part raw sex, in roughly equal amounts.

If Michelle and I flew to Paris and tried such a thing, we'd be arrested.

They'd void our passports, call us crazy Americans, and throw us out of their country, telling us never to come back.

But through the written word, we were able to enjoy that adventure risk-free.

Apparently I've had a secret obsession to run around a Parisian park late at night completely naked, swimming nude, and lying naked on a blanket under the stars.

Because hearing those words, and imagining the scene in my mind, turned me on tremendously.

And we were able to do it risk free.

No mosquitoes biting my butt. No strange fish nibbling on my penis as I swam. No gendarmes hauling our naked selves off to a holding cell.

Just Michelle and I doing in fantasy land what we'd never be able to do in real life.

It's quite nice. It really is.

But like I said, what stimulates me today might not work tomorrow.

When you shop for your erotica, be sure it's chock full of a variety of sexual adventures of all types.

From Michelle:

Here's a game you might consider playing which might help.

The Paris scene he's talking about went into great detail in the lovemaking scenes. When I was reading the part about the male character fondling and sucking on the female character's breasts, I put the book aside for a few minutes and offered Jacob the opportunity to suck on mine. Then I went back to reading. When I got to the part where the female character was performing oral sex on the male, I put the book aside and followed suit.

Doing this does two things... it actually puts him into the story and makes it easier to fantasize about it. And it makes it more exciting for him. Because unless we've done that particular scene so many times he's got it memorized, he doesn't know what's coming next.

He doesn't know whether the female character is going to climb atop him and insert him inside of her, or if the gendarmes are going to come running out of the bushes and slap them both into cuffs.

It's the not knowing what's next which help make the session more exciting and suspenseful.

As Jacob said, get a variety of erotica. It helps if you both pick it out together. Get something you can both enjoy, because like fighting ED, making love generally involves two people.

Okay, not always. But it's best when two people are involved.

Erectile Dysfunction Tool Box Thus Far: 5 Items

1. Frequent penis stimulation
2. Pin stimulation to penis head
3. Eat well. Diet is everything
4. Enlist your doctor's help
5. A good selection of written erotica

Chapter 7:   *You've Got to be Willing to Experiment in the Bedroom*

A Reminder: You promised to keep an open mind...

We have a lot of friends who are writers and journalists. That's to be expected, since that's our chosen profession.

After all, firemen tend to hang out with other firemen when they're off duty. Police officers tend to socialize with other police officers. Attorneys tend to associate with other attorneys, etc.

One of our closest writer friends is a guy we've known for years, since long before he got famous.

We'll call him "Al", which isn't his real name, but we promised to keep his name a secret when we wrote this book. You'll understand why in a minute.

Not long ago our friend was on a book tour which brought him within a hundred miles of our home, so he took a couple of days off, made a detour and came to visit.

It was during that visit he got a phone call from a friend, who tipped him off to something distressing.

The conversation that followed went something like this:

Al: My career is over.

Us: Why? What's happened?

Al: Remember Amy, the girl I broke up with a few months ago?

Us: Yes, we remember Amy. We always thought she was a real bitch.

Al: When we broke up my laptop disappeared. She said she didn't take it, but I always suspected she did.

Us: So? You can always get another laptop.

Al: You don't understand. The laptop had all the private videos we shot together.

Us: You mean private, as in… your own personal porn?

Al: Exactly. Amy plastered it all over the internet. The porn we made together, photos she took of me naked. Everything. I just got a call from another friend of mine. He's been watching the internet to see if any of it showed up. He said he went on line last night and Googled my name and added the word porn behind it.He said it's all over the internet. The porn, the pictures. Everything. My career is over, my life is ruined.

From Michelle:

For about two weeks we resisted the urge to go on Google and type in our friend's name.

I finally did it one night while Jacob was out because… well, I've always considered myself a curious sort.

Come on, ladies, back me up here. You've sometimes wondered about your male friends and what their dicks looked like, haven't you?

Surely I'm not the only one.

Ha! I thought so.

Anyway, it turned out that Al and Amy were quite adventurous in the bedroom.

Playful too.

I found a video of her playing "Whack A Mole" with his erect penis using a ping pong paddle which I found strangely erotic.

In another video she painted it with yellow fingernail polish and stuck a daisy in the end of it.

When Jacob came home I called him into my office and he stood over my shoulder while we perused the selection.

Some of them were just plain silly. In one, Amy told Al she always wanted a "black cock" and spray painted his dick and balls with a can of black spray paint.

In others, she videotaped him masturbating while watching porn on a laptop, or ejaculating while using a pink vibrator.

Our favorite was a video of her beating his dick with a stuffed chicken.

Yes, you read right. A stuffed chicken.

We called Al and asked him why a stuffed chicken. He said they used to come up with outrageous things to amuse themselves, not knowing that the videos would ever be made available for the world to see.

I told him I noticed his cock was hard as a rock in the videos. Since he's about our age, I asked him if he ever had trouble getting hard, or whether in the chicken video he was in his natural state.

He said he doesn't get as hard as easily as he once did, but that the videos were fun to shoot and he thoroughly enjoyed making them. He said he was especially aroused by the chicken and the ping pong paddle, and that he and Amy enjoyed very passionate lovemaking sessions after filming each of them.

That conversation, coincidentally, took place at the exact time Jacob and I were trying anything and everything to fix our ED problem.

So we said what the hell and went shopping for a stuffed chicken.

We couldn't find one, though, and had to settle for a teddy bear.

Al is a good friend of ours and a wonderful man, so we felt kind of bad at first to use his problems with his ex to help us in our battle over erectile dysfunction.

But he was very supportive of our decision. He only wanted the best for us, and recently told us he was glad his videos were able to entertain us, and to encourage us to experiment with such silly things ourselves.

That's the real contribution Al has given us. The ability to say, "Hey, that looks ridiculous, but it might be fun too."

Since watching Al's videos, Jacob and I have tried some silly things ourselves. None I want to discuss here, for they're our private guilty pleasures. And we didn't videotape them. We learned that much from Al's experience.

From Jacob:

The first of Amy and Al's videos we tried to duplicate was the ping pong paddle. She held my limp penis in the palm of her hand and tenderly whacked it a couple of times with the paddle.

I have to say going in that I felt absolutely ridiculous at first.

However... it turned out to be great fun. After just a few strokes with the paddle I was already hard. We stopped and made love and it was wonderful.

We've since added this particular activity to our ED tool box and use it occasionally. And we've learned some lessons from it.

First of all, ping pong paddles (at least the one we bought) come with two sides. One side has a rough texture and the other side is smooth.

Use the smooth side. The rough side can get a bit intense.

Don't overuse this method. Michelle paddles me only until I get hard and then we stop. We tried going longer one night and I was sore the next day.

Overall, though, it was silly, and it was fun. And it worked to make me hard.

It may or may not work for you too.

As for the stuffed chicken thing, we couldn't find a stuffed chicken. We bought a small brown teddy bear and tried it, in the same manner Amy used it on Al in their video.

It did nothing for me. But it was fun and silly and we laughed ourselves to sleep that night.

It's odd how certain things turn certain people on and yet doesn't do anything for the next guy.

But it also drives home a certain point. You never know until you try it what might give you an erection. That's why it's imperative you keep an open mind and be willing to try everything.

By the way Al, as we said, is a very good friend of ours. We asked his permission to use this particular story in our book project, and he gave us the okay.

For most of the last year, Al has tried to get the videos and photos Amy posted of him off the internet. But they were too widely spread, and getting them removed is a very long process.

He finally gave up and resolved himself to knowing that the whole world has seen him in his birthday suit, getting his wiener whacked with a stuffed chicken.

He says he's accepted it. His career didn't seem to suffer any damage after all. He says the only down side is that every time he meets someone new or someone asks him to sign one of his books for them he always wonders whether they've seen him naked.

And that sometimes he doesn't have to wonder. Sometimes they come right out and ask him about the chicken video.

We do feel bad for our good friend, but he is rather cavalier about the whole thing.

"I should have known better," he's quick to admit. "And I learned my lesson. No matter how much someone you love tells you they want to videotape you doing silly things to your wiener, don't believe her. I never will again."

So play. Experiment. Be silly and have some fun. You never know what might raise that sail and float your boat.

Just don't let anybody videotape it.

Erectile Dysfunction Tool Box Thus Far: 6 Items

1. Frequent penis stimulation
2. Pin stimulation to penis head
3. Eat well. Diet is everything
4. Enlist your doctor's help
5. A good selection of written erotica
6. Play. Experiment. Find new things to love

Chapter 8:   *Water is the most abundant resource on earth*

And believe it or not it can help with your ED problem

There are a myriad of things which can either cause erectile dysfunction, or contribute to its severity.

One of the most commonly overlooked of them is water.

Or rather, lack of same.

Specifically, the effects that mild dehydration upon the body can extend to your ability to get an erection. Really.

Our bodies cannot function without water. Other than oxygen, it's the single most important thing we need to keep us alive.

Even more than food.

That's why, stranded on a desert island, we'll die much faster from dehydration than from starvation.

That's also why doctors and dieticians have been telling us for a very long time to drink plenty of water. Because literally nothing in our bodies works right unless we're properly hydrated.

Sounds easy enough, doesn't it?

Doc: Drink more water.
You: Okay.

But when you walk out of the doctor's office it goes right out the window. You forego that glass of water because you're in a hurry and rush out the door. You could stop at that fast food place and get something to drink, but they're way too crowded. You could stop at the market a few blocks from your house and get something, but you're in a hurry to get home. There's that ball game coming on in just a few minutes, you see.

You could get up and get something to drink, but your team is getting ready to score.

Then the damned referee robs them of the score with a terrible call, and you're too angry to drink anything.

You're way too busy yelling at the TV.

Any of that sound familiar?

The fact is, very few of us intentionally drink water because we know it's good for us.

Nearly all of us wait to drink until we're thirsty.

And therein lies the problem.

For medical professionals will tell you that the very state of feeling thirsty is in itself a distress signal from our own bodies.

A distress signal which is saying, in effect, *"Hey dummy, you're neglecting me. I need water."*

Here's something that comes directly from the American Medical Association, and which might surprise you:

By the time you feel thirsty, you are **already** mildly dehydrated.

Thirst is, in effect, nature's alarm system. It's nature's way of saying our body is recognizing what we're ignoring.

It's the body's version of the "low fuel" light that lights up on your dashboard when you forget to stop at the 7-Eleven to fill up your tank.

Only this is more important, because we're not talking about a beat up old Chevy with a hanging bumper and a dent in the fender.

We're talking about your life here.

And while skipping that bottle of water or glass of iced tea will likely not kill you outright, mild dehydration can and will affect your body in a lot of ways. And over the long term, it can cause very serious problems.

Like shorten the lives of some of your vital organs.

Okay, enough talking of generalities. Let's get into specifics.

Mild dehydration makes it harder for your body to process the food you eat. It takes moisture to force that stuff through your intestinal tract. Moisture for your stomach to break it down. Moisture to push the waste from your body. It makes your internal organs, pretty much all of them, work harder to do their jobs. And theoretically, shortening their lives before they start to wear out.

The problem is, even the experts can't agree on how much water you should drink to stay healthy. Some say eight eight ounce glasses per day. For those of you who failed math as I did that's...

Hold on a minute while I ask Michelle.

Okay, that's half a gallon a day. Sixty four ounces. That, in our estimation, is reasonable, as long as it includes the coffee we drink in the morning and the Dr. Pepper we suck down with our lunch. And those two Budweisers we drink while we're watching the ball game after dinner.

Ah, but there's the rub.

Many experts say that sixty four ounces isn't enough. Some say we need twice that much. Others say we need three times that much.

We don't know about you, but the idea of someone placing a gallon and a half of liquid on our dining room table and telling us we have to drink it all before we go to bed that night is a little bit daunting.

Or maybe impossible.

To make the problem worse, many of the experts now say that caffeinated beverages shouldn't count. They've known for quite some time that caffeine can actually dry out our system. More on that in a bit.

Still other experts say that alcoholic beverages shouldn't count.

But if we cut out the coffee, and the soft drinks, and the beer, what's left?

Just water. Plain, boring water.

If you're like us, you don't mind downing a couple of bottles of drinking water every day. There's nothing better to quench your thirst on a hot day.

But downing twenty bottles a day to make some of the experts happy is a bit much.

Luckily, not all of the experts discount those types of drinks. We like those experts better.

You might be asking what water and dehydration have to do with erectile dysfunction.

That's because mild dehydration can inhibit your penis's ability to stand up and do those things you like to do with it.

Really.

You see, water does something else besides keep your organs working at peak capacity. It also lubricates the blood which courses through your body and into your penis to make it erect. When your body is dehydrated, the blood thickens. Yes, the change is slight and subtle. And slightly thickened blood doesn't really affect most of your other bodily functions.

But it can restrict blood flow to your penis.

And it's the blood flow, my friends, which make your penis hard and makes your wife happy.

You see, your penis consists largely of tiny blood vessels which contract when it's flaccid and expand when blood flows into them.

Because the vessels are so tiny, thickened blood has a harder time getting into them. And if the blood can't get into them the penis won't get as hard.

The early bird may get the worm,
but the thin blood gets the dick hard.

Remember that. It may sound silly because, well… because it is. But if remembering it will help remind you to drink plenty of water, especially on the days you expect to dally in the bedroom later, then it'll serve its purpose.

Let's conduct a little experiment to drive this point home before we leave it and go on to something else.

And you can do the experiment in your mind if you wish. It's far less messy that way.

Say you take a regular garden hose and lay one end on the ground. Hold the other end about waist high.

This hose represents just one of the blood vessels in your penis. The ones which carry blood to the penis and make it hard (and there are hundreds of them).

Take a pitcher of water and pour it into the hose. Watch how fast the water flows through it.

Then take a pitcher of maple syrup and do the same thing.

See the difference?

Apply that to your blood. Well-lubricated blood in a body that's well hydrated will have a much easier time filling those tiny vessels in your penis. And you'll have a much easier time getting and maintaining your erection.

Seriously.

From Jacob:

Back in my Army days I was stationed at Fort Irwin, California, on the edge of the high desert.

My folks lived in Texas then, just outside of Dallas. This was before I met and fell in love with Michelle. I was single, young and stupid.

And I had a brand spanking new F-150 pickup.

No one feels more invincible than a young soldier in an F-150 pickup.

Looking back now, I know it was a stupid thing to do. But back then I had a different mindset. A devil-may-care attitude. A bunch of rocks in my head.

I drove from Ft. Irwin to Dallas at least three times a year. I got thirty days leave, and normally went for ten days at a time.

Some of my buddies gave me a hard time about spending all my leave to hang out with my parents. I didn't care. I loved them. I wish I had them back. And besides, there was plenty of time on the weekends or down days to go hunting and fishing with my friends.

I know now that thirty days of leave per year is a rather generous amount. But back then I saw it as not enough. To me it was a precious commodity and I hated to waste a single minute of it.

The Army had a regulation that said when you were on leave you couldn't travel more than four hundred miles per day. That was to keep soldiers from falling asleep at the wheel and killing themselves. It wasn't necessarily that the Army cared much about us. But they spent a lot of time training us, and if one of us dumb clucks went and killed ourselves they had to start all over and train someone else to take our place.

I actually had a first sergeant who told me that.

The Army was so filled with love.

The same first sergeant told me that if I was stupid enough to die in a car crash on his watch, that he would personally beat my ass.

"I don't care if you're in a dozen pieces. I will super glue you back together just so I can tear you apart again."

As I said, back then I had my own way of doing things, Army regulations be damned.

The way I figured it, if I only drove four hundred miles per day, it would take me two and a half days to get there. It would also take me two and a half days to drive back.

That's five days. That's half my leave time. I didn't want to spend half my leave time on the road.

On top of that, I'd have had to stay at a roadside motel for two nights each way. That was two hundred bucks on an E-4's pay.

And I was an incredible cheapskate. That wouldn't do either.

I was fortunate in that my unit never asked to see motel receipts for soldiers returning from long drives. Some of the other units did that, but mine never did.

That was a godsend, for it allowed me to drive 2300 miles from Fort Irwin to my mom and dad's house, stopping only for gasoline.

I didn't even stop to eat. To save money I made a dozen baloney and cheese sandwiches, on white bread with mustard.

I put them on top of a layer of ice in a big cooler that rode on the seat in front of me.

Whenever I was hungry, I reached over and popped the lid on the cooler and took out a sandwich. When I got thirsty I reached beneath the ice and took out a bottle of Dr. Pepper.

Dr. Pepper was my best friend back in those days. I sucked them down like some of my friends sucked down beer.

At night I merely pulled my truck over on the side of the road to urinate. In the daytime I watched for the roadside rest areas and peed there whenever I could. When there wasn't one in sight I pulled over and filled up one of my empty Dr. Pepper bottles, then disposed of it in the nearest roadside litter barrel.

It was a hell of a way to travel, but my logic was sound. At least in my own feeble mind it was.

If I did things the Army way I'd have had five days to spend at home with my parents and my old high school friends.

If I bucked the system and did things my own rebellious way I had eight days. Those three extra days were what drove me.

Yes, I was exhausted when I finally made it home.

And yes, when I finally got some sleep I generally slept for a lot of hours. And yes, I was a cranky son of a bitch for the first two days I was back.

But none of that mattered to me.

The one adverse affect my marathon drive did was cause me to lose my voice.

It happened every single time. Winter or summer, it didn't matter. By the time I got to Dallas my throat was raw. I could barely get out a squeak. I learned to communicate in a very loud whisper. It was painful to do that, but at least my voice didn't crack and only allow me to speak every tenth word.

I was baffled. My mom was worried. My younger sister, still living at home while she went to college, was pleased. My being unable to speak gave her much more time to rattle on and on about nothing.

The same thing happened upon my return to Ft. Irwin. My first two days I'd lose my voice for no apparent reason.

No one in my family had ever suffered from laryngitis.

So we ruled that out.

Mom was convinced I was allergic to something. But they still lived in the same house I grew up with, with the same flowers in her garden and the same pollens in the air. And it seemed too odd a coincidence that my allergy attacks were coordinated so nicely with the first two days of my visit. It didn't matter whether it was winter or summer. And in my whole time at Fort Irwin, I never so much as sneezed. But I lost my voice the first two days I came back from leave.

Every time, without fail.

The mystery was finally solved when my supervisor said I was no good to him as a mime.

"Report to the infirmary and get some medicine. And goddamn it, you'd better be talking when you come back."

Everybody knew that the doctors weren't allowed to rat you out. Even if they were aware you broke some kind of rules to injure yourself, they had to follow the doctor-patient privilege and keep it to themselves.

That's the only reason I was straight with him.

That and the whole losing my voice thing was driving me crazy.

Doc: So, you say you just got back from leave?
Me (whispering): Yes sir.
Doc: Where'd you go?
Me: A little town just south of Dallas.

Doc: Could be the air on your airplane. It's recycled, and very dry. You might have picked up somebody else's bug, or the dry air might have dried out your throat. Did you sleep with your mouth open on the flight?

Me: I didn't fly, sir. I drove.

I remember him scratching his chin, just like they do in the movies.

Doc: I see. Has it ever happened before?

Me: Yes, sir. Every time I drive home on leave. And every time I drive back here.

I could almost see the light come on in his eyes.

Doc: Let me guess. You drove straight through.

Me (sheepishly): Yes sir.

Doc: How long does that take you?

Me: Right at twenty three hours if the roads are dry and traffic is light.

He whistled under his breath.

Doc: That's a lot of hours. What did you take to stay awake? You didn't get any speed from a trucker, did you?

Me: No sir. I may not be real smart, but I know better than to use drugs. I drank Dr. Pepper the whole way.

Doc: And how many Dr. Peppers did you drink, exactly?

Me: I got two six packs before I left and drank them all.

Doc: I see (he said "I see" a lot. The sucker must have had perfect vision.)

Doc: Were they cans or bottles?
Me: Bottles.
Doc. I see. That's a lot of soda.
Me: Yes sir.
Doc: And that's what's causing you to lose your voice.
Me: Pardon me?
Doc: Caffeine does terrible things to the human body. One of them that isn't well known is that it dries out the vocal cords.
Me: Wow! Seriously?
Doc: Seriously.
Me: I see.

I learned a serious lesson that day. First of all, that caffeine does terrible things to the human body. Some of them, like increased blood pressure and gastrointestinal problems, are well known. Others, like the vocal cord thing, took me by complete surprise.

And here's a bigger surprise: According to my good friend Paul, who is also my doctor, there have been studies which appear to link caffeine use with... you guessed it. Erectile Dysfunction.

Okay, I rambled a bit. I tend to do that sometimes when I write. But I did have a point.

For your body (including your penis) to work properly, you must stay well hydrated. But there's a right way to hydrate yourself and a wrong way. Drinking way too much soda or coffee is the wrong way.

Remember I mentioned earlier that even the experts can't agree about how much water we should drink every day?

I'm going to give you a valuable tip, and a rule of thumb to tell whether you're adequately hydrated.

It's one of only two things I learned during my stint in the United States Army (the first was the vocal cord thing).

When I was at Fort Irwin, we went into the field several times a year.

Going into the field is like a big camping trip, only it's not fun.

Since Fort Irwin was on the edge of the high desert, we had a problem with guys falling out from dehydration. Their bodies grew weak and they just passed out.

To add to the problem, nobody took any real effort to make sure we drank enough. Keeping track of how much water every soldier drank would have been a nightmare.

And to be honest, the amount they needed varied. For example, in the winter months we didn't sweat and needed less.

It the hot days of summer we sweated buckets and needed up to three times more water.

Nobody ever died from it. At least not while I was there. We simply took those soldiers and found a shady spot to lie them in, then cooled them off by dousing them with water.

Our lieutenant wouldn't let them stand up until they drank two liters of water.

Okay, I'm rambling again.

Here's the second thing I learned in the Army.

Our first sergeant taught us to evaluate the degree of our hydration not by the amount of water we drank...

... but by the color of our pee.

You see, your pee should be clear. Every time you go, except for first thing in the morning. That's because you've gone all night long without drinking.

First thing in the morning it's permissible for your urine to be yellow. But you should start tanking up on water and a limited amount of carbonated or caffeinated beverages right after that. So that the next time you urinate the stream is clear.

And you should urinate at least five times a day. If you're not, you're not taking in enough fluid.

Hey, that's three things I learned, not two.

God bless the United States Army.

Erectile Dysfunction Tool Box Thus Far: 8 Items

1. Frequent penis stimulation
2. Pin stimulation to penis head
3. Eat well. Diet is everything
4. Enlist your doctor's help
5. A good selection of written erotica
6. Play. Experiment. Find new things to love
7. Water is our friend. Drink lots of it.
8. Limit caffeine

Chapter 9:   *A few words about all those items you've been adding to your toolbox*

And how they're going to help you...

Men are like snowflakes for two reasons. First, because they melt in the warm hands of the woman they love.

But mostly because no two are alike.

They all have their own tastes when it comes to food, fashion, women, and a myriad of other things.

Bearing that in mind, it should come to no one's surprise that what works with one man might not work with another.

This is most notably true of medications. The reason your doctor might try you on several different medications before deciding on which one to treat you with is because some medications simply work better on some people than on others.

Michelle found this out when she went in to be treated for gastritis.

The first thing her doctor gave her was the most popular drug on the market. "It works well for most people," her doctor told her.

But it made Michelle even worse. The second medication seemed to help, but the dry mouth and sleepiness Michelle suffered as side effects made it not worth the benefits.

The third medication was, as they say, the charm. She started taking it about two years ago and it's worked wonders.

Okay, why are we talking about Michelle's gastritis instead of erectile dysfunction?

Simply to drive home this point:

The tools in our own personal toolbox, which solved our ED problem, might not work quite as well for you.

That's why you need to put as many things in your toolbox as possible. So that if you discard some of them outright, or you try some of them and find they don't work for you, you still have other options.

Also, and we cannot stress this enough, you must keep an open mind.

Here's why:

Some of you may say, "I'm not going to try that particular option. It's stupid. And I don't think I'd like it."

Remember when your kid told you he didn't want to play soccer because he thought it was stupid and he wouldn't like it? And you talked him into signing up for a youth league anyway, with the promise that if he didn't like it he could drop it after the first season?

Remember when that same kid decided he loved it? And that he was a three year varsity player in high school and got an athletic scholarship to his college of choice?

The same thing could happen to you. You could decide not to try something because it makes you feel uncomfortable or feel it's beneath you.

And you might find that not only do you like it after all. But that it's the one item in your toolbox that works best for you.

That's why you must keep an open mind, and why we'll keep preaching on that until the end of this book.

It's also why we're going to pump as many tools into your toolbox as we can. Because some won't work in your particular situation and will be discarded. Some will work well one night, but not at all the next night. (Don't discard those).

And some, we're betting, will work for you.

The more arrows in your quiver, the more likely you are to win the battle. The more wrenches in your garage, the more likely you are to fix your car.

And the more tools in your ED toolbox, the more likely you are to conquer it.

From Michelle:

I've always been very open and upfront with my thoughts and actions. To be honest, it's cost me an occasional friend. I'm the type of person who, if you have a booger hanging from your nose, will tell you you have a booger hanging from your nose.

Many of your friends won't mention it to you, either because it embarrasses them, or for fear it might embarrass you. So they won't say anything, and will let you walk around the mall while people snicker at you behind your back.

I contend friends like that aren't truly your friends at all.

Jacob and I had a theory when we were working our "Ed" project.

(Yes, we actually gave our project a human name, so we could say, at a cocktail party, "We should consider that for Ed" and people wouldn't necessarily know what we were talking about)

Our theory was that many of our friends might also be silently suffering from the same issues we were, as many of them are our same age or older.

Men are hard headed and stubborn, and intensely proud. They're very unlikely to admit to their friends they're having erectile problems.

Too many of them view it as a loss of their manhood, a reduction of their virility.

They're big dummies.

If they spoke of it frankly with their friends, and found out which of their friends were also suffering, and traded ideas like women exchange recipes, there'd be no reason for us to have to write this book.

But most men can't bring themselves to do that.

So I took the initiative, and I'd encourage you ladies to do the same.

I brought up the subject first with my best friend Stacy over an afternoon lunch. I didn't want to put her on the defensive, or imply her own husband was having problems with intimacy. And at the same time, I knew she was one of those women who loves it when someone shares secrets with her.

She's very good at keeping secrets too. Which is why I started with her.

By the way, Stacy isn't her real name. She gave me permission to use this in the book, provided I didn't use her real name. She was concerned that it might embarrass her husband Tom (not his real name either)

Anyway, as I said I was very careful in the way I approached the subject.

I said, "If I tell you something extremely personal, can you keep it a secret?"

As I suspected, she gave me her rapt attention and said, "Sure!"

Me: We're having problems in the bedroom lately. Jacob's having problems getting hard and staying that way

Stacy: Oh, my goodness. I'm so sorry to hear that. What are you doing for it?

Me: He went to see Paul, his doctor, last week. Paul gave him some ideas, and we've been doing a lot of research on the internet.

Stacy: Did his doctor prescribe some medication?

Me: He offered, but we decided we want to use that as a last resort. He told Jacob there are a lot of other methods which might work for us that don't involve medication.

Stacy: Have you tried ice cubes and warming oils?

Me (somewhat taken aback): Pardon me?

Stacy: I'm telling you this only because I know I can trust you to keep it to yourself. But Tom has problems too sometimes.

Me: Do tell...

Stacy: Sometimes when he's having trouble getting hard I'll get up and go to the kitchen and get an ice cube. I'll put it in my mouth and go down on him. Something about the combination of my warm mouth and the coldness from the ice cube seems to turn him on just enough to make him hard.

Me: I never thought of that. We'll have to add that to our toolbox.

Stacy: It doesn't always work. But it frequently does. You might also try warming oils.

Me: Tell me more.

Stacy: There are several brands on the market. K-Y has a good one. That's the one we use. But if you don't like that one there are several others. They're available at drug stores and are on the shelf so you don't have to ask for them. Also, I think Walmart carries them as well.

Me: We've never used them. Are they specifically made for ED?

Stacy: No. Actually, they're sexual lubricants, for women who have lubrication issues. But they actually warm up in your hands, and on your husband's penis, and in Tom's case actually acts as a stimulant. He enjoys the warmth of it, and sometimes all it takes is me playing with him with the oil on my hands to make him hard.

Me: Sold! We'll try it.

Stacy: Of course, it doesn't work for all men. I have another friend from my old job whose husband was having the same problem, and I suggested it. She said he also enjoyed the warmth, but didn't get hard from it. In other words, it doesn't work on all peni.

Me: Peni?

Stacy: Sure. Peni. If the plural of cactus is cacti, then isn't the plural of penis peni?

Me: Okay, now you're just plain nuts.

Stacy: Possibly. But try those two things and see if they work.

We did indeed try those two things. The ice cube did nothing for Jacob at all. He didn't like the sensation of the cold on his dick. He said dicks were supposed to seek out warm places, not cold ones.

Good point, and different strokes for different folks.

The warming oils had mixed results for us. We got a bottle of the K-Y version at our local Walmart, off the shelf without having to talk to a pharmacist.

It worked wonderfully well the first time we tried it. Jacob laid back as I massaged his dick with the oil, his eyes rolled to the back of his head. He obviously enjoyed it. He was hard in a couple of minutes and we made love. I must say it was very enjoyable to me as well.

The second time we tried it, nothing. The third time it worked again.

And that brings up another point. What works one night might not work another night. Never ever ever (did I mention never) throw away one of the items in your toolbox because it didn't work or because you're too squeamish to try it. On another night you might be more open-minded and ready to try new things, or you might have better luck with something which failed you before.

We're adding both these items to your toolbox. Just because the ice cube method didn't work for us doesn't necessarily mean it won't work for you.

Erectile Dysfunction Tool Box Thus Far: 10 Items

1. Frequent penis stimulation
2. Pin stimulation to penis head
3. Eat well. Diet is everything
4. Enlist your doctor's help
5. A good selection of written erotica
6. Play. Experiment. Find new things to love
7. Water is our friend. Drink lots of it.
8. Limit caffeine
9. Ice can be nice
10. Try warming oils as a stimulant

Chapter 10:   *Pay attention, this one's important.*

Don't overlook the power of a visual stimulant

Mention the word "pornography" to anyone, and you'll typically get a strong response.

Although it's certainly more accepted now than it once was, especially on the internet, women as a whole still tend to view it as dirty.

Men as a whole, though, are either indifferent to it or love it. Many men would never get on their computers, except to search for porn.

In our particular situation, we chose to look upon it as a possible means to help fix our ED problem. And in that regard, it helped us at least as much as anything else we tried.

Those people who study such things have known for years that women are more stimulated by the erotic word. Men are more stimulated by visual erotica.

The same studiers of such things never could really agree on why, although the prevailing theory is a time factor. When women read erotica they aren't in a hurry. They like to cozy up to a good book and read it at length. Not necessarily to masturbate, although some of them do. But mostly to visualize themselves in the story and to escape the realities of their hum-drum sex life for a time.

Most men, on the other hand, use visual porn as a masturbation tool. Sometimes they envision themselves as the man in the video rolling around in bed with a beautiful woman. More often than not, though, they merely use that beautiful woman and her actions as a way to stimulate themselves and obtain an erection. That, in turn, enables them to masturbate while watching her.

For men, porn is simply a means to an end. And while a woman can read a good erotica book for hours, men generally want to get the deed done and get it over with. It's a matter of expediency.

Our own personal theory: this explains why men's tastes in porn are different than women's. Women, when they shop for porn, are looking for something with a storyline. Something that provides a bit of entertainment between the sex sessions. Something that makes it a bit more like the erotica books they prefer.

Men, on the other hand, couldn't care less about the plot of the movie. In fact, for most of them, the only plot is the actors and actresses crawling into bed and knocking their knees together.

The effect (or possible effect) on your ED problem, though, is something not in dispute.

Studies have shown that even at an advanced age (men over 60), visual porn can stimulate a man more than erotica, more than physical stimulation alone, more even than some of the ED medication.

But… and here's the rub… you have to know how to use it.

Guys, if you leave your wife waiting in the bedroom while you run off to another room to watch porn and make yourself hard, you're likely to lose that erection shortly after you return to your wife.

That's not good. For one thing, it defeats the purpose of even having the porn. For another, it's very likely to reinforce any feelings of inadequacy your wife may have. In the back of her mind she may worry that she's not as attractive or exciting as that much-younger woman on the TV or computer screen.

And that will certainly do nothing to help your ED problem.

We recommend moving the porn into the bedroom with you. To play on your television in the background during foreplay, and continuing all the way through your lovemaking session.

Michelle has discussed this with enough of her friends to get the sense the wives would be more opposed to this than their husbands. And to be sure, it is rather disconcerting for a wife to watch her husband gain an erection while watching younger women have sex. Especially when she herself was unable to help him maintain an erection a few minutes before.

We understand that. We get it. It's a big psychological barrier for women to invite other women into the bedroom to help stimulate their husbands.

But here's where the whole "open mind" thing comes in.

If the wife can overcome that hurdle, visual porn can be one of, if not the, most effective tool in your toolbox.

And remember, ladies, he doesn't get hard because he'd prefer to make love to the woman on the screen than you. He gets hard because, well, men are wired differently when it comes to sex. For millions of years, sex for women was merely a means to procreate, to further the species. It was a key ticket to pregnancy and childbirth. The orgasm was merely a reward to encourage women to have sex. Whether you believe in evolution or in a greater power, that much is not in dispute.

Men, however, don't get pregnant or have babies. For men, the only real purpose for having sex is to feel good. And as such, he's generally more apt to want to get it started and get it done. That's why he's aroused much more quickly than women, And it's also why he's stimulated by things which don't always stimulate the woman.

Whether you like it or not, for the vast majority of men, pornography is stimulating to some degree.

And for a lot of men who have erectile dysfunction it is the only thing which works.

Studies have shown that watching pornography while stimulating the penis is the most effective way of obtaining an erection for almost ninety percent of men. And it's the second most effective method for men suffering from moderate ED, after medicinal means (which we'll talk about soon)

So, then, let's recap.

- Playing with the penis, either by its owner or by proxy (wife), makes the penis hard
- Nearly all men have used porn to masturbate at some point in their lives
- Many married men still use porn to masturbate occasionally, mostly for reasons of expediency
- While many women find porn dirty or icky, most men are okay with it.
- PORN IS ONE OF THE BEST TOOLS IN YOUR TOOLBOX. DON'T IGNORE IT.

Of course, before you can use it, you wives are going to get past the ickiness of it all. (Our spell-check says that word doesn't exist. That's because we just made it up)

Anyway, you get our point. If you wives (or girlfriends or significant others) can get past the stigma of using porn as a tool, it can usually help at least a little. And it can frequently help a lot.

From Michelle:

I'll admit I was one of those women who thought pornography was a bit on the shady side. I think it's because of the way society views it. Society tends to adopt a holier-than-thou attitude when it comes to pornography, placing it just below prostitution. It intentionally ignores the fact that society's mayors, police chiefs, clergy and educators are mostly males, and as such, are just as likely as any other male to whack their wienie every once in a while.

And let's face it, the majority of them are watching some type of pornography while they're tugging away on that little fella.

I guess my biggest hang-up regarding pornography was that I viewed it as pointless. I mean, it did nothing for me. Or very little, anyway. I thought it was interesting to a degree. I mean, it showed me that all penises were not alike (or pussies, for that matter) and I saw some things I wanted to try with Jacob.

But it didn't turn me on.

But then again, I'm not a man.

I've known for quite some time that men are stimulated in different ways than women. They're way more visual than we are.

Women, on the other hand, are much more likely to be stimulated sexually by the written word. I guess that's why I've always been more apt to get in the mood by reading a romance novel heavy on the erotica, while Jacob was more likely to be turned on by watching the cheerleaders at the football game.

But I tried to keep an open mind because, by all accounts, pornography can be a very effective tool to correct ED.

Going in, I asked Jacob what, in his view, pornography meant to the average male.

"When you see that hot twenty year old blonde with the impossibly big tits sucking on that guy's dick, do you wish it was you? Do you wish I looked like her? Do you wish you could trade me in on someone who looked like her?"

He assured me that wasn't the case. And he was sincere.

"When men masturbate to porn, it's merely a way to accomplish a mission," he said. "It doesn't mean I don't still find you beautiful. It doesn't mean I don't love you any less than I ever did. And it certainly doesn't mean I want the twenty year old blonde. God no!"

That made me feel better.

And for the record, I've never been opposed to the whole porn thing. I was just indifferent to it.

But when we read from several reliable sources it could be used to aid in ED, I quickly became a fan.

I should point out that we use it not as most men use porn. Most men go off to their bedroom when their wife isn't around, turn on the porn, pull out that little sucker and abuse it until it squirts.

That's NOT how to use it effectively to help your ED.

The correct way to use it is to have it on in the bedroom (on a television. A typical computer monitor isn't large enough to see from the bed and is therefore worthless). It is an accompaniment to your lovemaking, not the main feature.

In other words, it's merely on in the background for you guys to watch while you and the wife are doing other things to give you an erection. Even after you're hard and making love to your wife, an occasional glance can help keep you hard.

Some things to remember, for both of you:

Guys, although the porn is mainly for your benefit, it's much nicer when your lady enjoys it too. Pick out some that has attractive men in it as well as attractive women. The best option is for the two of you to pick it out together.

Also, guys, be discrete. Don't make it obvious if you're focusing a considerable amount of attention to the television while you're getting aroused. It's okay to do it. After all, that's the whole purpose of even using the porn. Just don't make it obvious. Watching discretely is acceptable. Yelling, "Look at the tits on that babe..." is not. Be respectful of your wife and her feelings.

And always, always, always, focus your attention on your wife once you're hard and ready to go. She's the one who loves you. She's the one who tolerates all your foolishness. She's the one you want to please, not some bimbo on the TV screen.

Ladies, keep an open mind. This is mostly for him, but if you watch it with an open mind you might enjoy it too. Most women aren't turned on by visual porn, but then again a surprising number of them are. Insist on helping him pick it out so it's something both of you might enjoy. You'll find it a lot more palatable that way.

Ladies, when you pick out the porn, try to go light on the storyline. A lot of modern porn has tried to get away from the wall-to-wall sex scenes in recent years and has actually included plotlines or storylines. It's been done in an effort to lure more women customers.

The thinking was that if they made the videos more entertaining, more like soap operas, women might be more apt to buy them and watch them. The sex was and always will be the primary focus. But it's not always the only focus.

At least for some porn movies

*The problem is, it's not the storyline which "raises the sail" on your husband's boat. So try to be a bit understanding if **he** wants more sex and less acting.*

From Jacob:

Once we decided to include pornography in our toolbox, we set some guidelines.

We ruled out internet porn outright for several reasons.

Mostly because downloading internet porn sites is undisputedly the number one way to put viruses and malware on your computer. And since both of us make our living using our computers, that wouldn't be good.

Also, the logistics of using porn from the internet is difficult.

For example, the movies you download from a porn site are typically in MP-4 format. They can be played on a computer, but not on a television set. And as Michelle mentioned earlier, a tiny computer monitor halfway across the room is not conducive for our needs.

In other words, if I can't even see it without my glasses (and I always take my glasses off for sex) then why even bother?

The solution, for us, was a visit to the local "Adult Store."

By the way, they're called "Novelty Stores" in some cities. But whatever it's called, your city has them. And if you feel squeamish about going into them, don't be. The stigma of frequenting such places went away years ago. These days you're more likely to see someone you know from church or work than seeing a seedy guy in a trench coat.

Most adult stores will allow you to rent the movies before you actually purchase them. We recommend you do that, since it's sometimes hard to tell from the box whether it'll meet your needs. Rental fees are typically five to seven dollars for a forty-eight hour period. A typical video sells from $59 to $89, depending on the quality and content.

Before Michelle and I went in we agreed on the process we'd use.

Since the whole purpose of the thing was to help me get and maintain an erection, we focused on things I liked. Pretty girls doing sexy things to their guys and vice versa.

At the same time, we recognized that it should be pleasing to Michelle too. So we gave her "veto authority."

I agreed that if she didn't think she'd find the video pleasing, she could shoot it down for any reason. It was the least I could do to appease her. After all, it's a big thing for a woman to accept that her husband is getting turned on by watching other women.

Initially I selected seven videos to rent and take home. Some had storylines and some didn't. Some were just ninety minutes of raw, unadulterated sex.

She shot down three of them. One, she said, just looked too "trashy," whatever that meant. She shot down one because all the men on the back cover were ugly and unappealing. The third one se didn't like because the main actress looked too much like a girl I was dating when Michelle and I first met. I didn't even realize it until she pointed it out, and I haven't seen the woman in thirty years, but okay. A deal was a deal.

We rented the four and watched them over the course of two nights.

We took two of them back and purchased the other two.

From Michelle:

Remember, these are a tool for you to use in conjunction with other tools. The porn is not a means unto itself to achieve an erection.

And we don't always use the porn, either. One of the most important things you can do to get that erection on a regular basis is to use a variety of things. If you use the same methods every time, they'll become humdrum and routine and will stop working.

I'd say we use the porn roughly half the time.

When we do use it, we put the DVD in and play it in the background, on the 42 inch television in the corner of our bedroom.

Jacob can see it while we play, but I typically have my back to it while I'm doing some of the other things we already talked about.

I think it's the combination of several different stimuli which make this method effective. They build on one another.

My gently sucking on his penis and massaging his balls might not by itself make him hard.

By my doing that while he's watching the porn on TV might do the trick.

While he's watching it, I'll try several of the other methods until we find one that works.

About eighty five to ninety percent of the time we're successful in getting him hard. When it works, we typically tune out the TV and make love like we always have.

The other ten to fifteen percent, the times we can't get him hard, we do other things instead. One thing I love about Jacob is he never leaves me high and dry. He's always said he enjoys giving me an orgasm as much as having one himself, and he's proved it time and time again.

There have been several times when we've started out with him watching the women on the video, trying to get hard. And then we've ended up with him going down on me while I watched the men on the video.

Turnabout, as they say, is fair play.

From Jacob:

A couple of final notes before we let this one go:

You'll have to decide what to do about the sound. The actresses in these kinds of films are paid to scream loudly during their sex scenes. The screaming may be offensive to some, since they frequently have what we used to call "potty mouth" when our kids were small.

Or, the sound may be a distraction when you're trying to do other stuff.

For me personally, the sound is a bit of a turn-on and helps me stay erect when Michelle and I are making love, even when I can't see the screen because I'm busy doing other things.

It may, therefore, be a bit of a turn-on for some of you guys as well.

We leave the sound on both during foreplay, (when we're working on making my little friend hard) and leave it on while we're making love. But we keep it at a relatively low volume, so that it enhances the session without overpowering it.

Think background music, but it's not music...

If that doesn't work for you, simply mute the sound, but leave the TV on as a visual assist for your guy.

Also, we've found that after a few months of using the same videos over and over again they lose some of its effect.

No, I don't know why. I mean, I certainly haven't tired of seeing Michelle's body for all these years. But I've tired of seeing the same bodies time and time again on the television.

Perhaps it's because I'm not madly and deeply in love with the actresses on the screen, as I am with Michelle.

Anyway, the same thing may or may not happen to you, guys.

If it does, plan on refreshing your porn every few months.

Not all adult stores offer trade-in credit, but the one we go to does. In fact, that's one of the reasons we go there. When we trade in a video we're tired of we get a thirty percent credit back on it.

If your store doesn't offer return credit, you might try some of your other guy friends to see if they'd be willing to trade.

You'd be surprised how many of your guy friends have impressive collections of porn.

What? You thought you were the only one who masturbated ferociously when you were a kid, and who still does so occasionally?

Au contraire, my friend. Au contraire.

That's French for "on the contrary."

Or, in other terms you may understand: No way, Jose.

Most men masturbate. Even the people you work with, your neighbors, your clergy. Your boss, although that visual may be too much for you to think of.

And while it might be just a bit disturbing to think of your minister masturbating, he likely does, and probably did a lot when he was younger.

Of course, if you're too shy to brooch the subject and ask your friends if they have any porn to trade (we can certainly understand why you wouldn't want to ask your minister), your adult store isn't far away.

And if you don't have an adult store close by, you can order adult DVDs off the internet.

Just don't download videos on your computer. It'll almost guarantee your computer becomes infected with viruses.

Erectile Dysfunction Tool Box Thus Far: 11 Items

1. Frequent penis stimulation
2. Pin stimulation to penis head
3. Eat well. Diet is everything
4. Enlist your doctor's help
5. A good selection of written erotica
6. Play. Experiment. Find new things to love
7. Water is our friend. Drink lots of it.
8. Limit caffeine
9. Ice can be nice
10. Try warming oils as a stimulant
11. Porn as a visual mood setter

Chapter 10: *Using Viagra and Cialis to supplement your efforts*

And some tips on how best to use them.

Many doctors are quick to prescribe Cialis and Viagra and send their patients on their happy way.

Many patients walk out of their doctors' offices with big smiles on their faces, thinking their problems are permanently solved.

They are great medications, both of them. Although they use two different methods to help with your ED, they're both quite affective for most men. But just like every other medication, they do have side effects. Before taking them, therefore, you must listen to your doctor's warnings, or to what they say in their commercials.

We should also say that the companies which make these two medications are on the up and up. They're honest with you from the beginning about possible side effects and don't try to hide them, as many other products tend to do.

You know which ones we're talking about. The commercials which start out by screaming,

COME TO OUR CAR DEALERSHIP. WE'LL GIVE YOU FIVE THOUSAND DOLLARS OFF ON THIS PARTICULAR MODEL!

And then, in tiny words they flash briefly at the bottom of the screen, in a color meant to blend into the background to make it even more difficult to read, it explains further:

There is no way, no how, we're gonna give you anything off of this model or any other. We'll pretend to, but what we'll actually do is jack up your interest rate so you pay more than the five thousand dollars, and at the same time we'll reduce what we give you for your trade in. Because we consider you a sucker and we are always looking for new ways to fleece you. And oh, by the way, we had only one left in that particular model and it's long gone. But here's a better model you can't really afford but which gives us a higher commission...

The commercials for Viagra and Cialis are, on the other hand, totally legitimate. They don't try to deceive you by underplaying the possible side effects. They lay them out so you can make an informed decision as to whether their products are right for you.

But it's still very important stuff, and you need to listen and consider it. Just as you would for any other medication.

Now, having said that, we have nothing against either Viagra or Cialis. They are great things, which help many men across every country in the world. And there are certain side effects and risks with virtually every prescription drug. So we're not advocating against them. We're simply making the same recommendation we'd make if you were considering any other drug. Make sure you consider the possible side effects.

From Jacob:

Paul, my doctor and one of my best friends, ran a battery of tests on me before agreeing to let me try Viagra. He wanted to make sure my heart was strong enough to handle it, and also considered whether the increased sexual activity would be too hard on my old body.

I assured him I was in good shape for a man of my age.

He gave me a "side eye" and said "being able to lift a bottle of beer from the bar to your mouth several times in the same hour does not mean you're in shape."

I reminded him that I play golf at least two mornings a week. And that I occasionally finish before the sun sets.

He said, "You gotta do better than that."

I told him he was just pissed off because I beat him in bowling last weekend. And then I reminded him I walk a mile or so with Michelle every day.

He still wasn't impressed.

But he finally relented after he made me pee into a bottle, donate what seemed like a gallon of my blood and put me on a treadmill.

Then he asked what my sexual habits were.

Me: Well, I don't fuck goats, if that's what you're asking.

Him: Are you sure?

Me: Well, there was that one time when I was in college. But I was lonely back then. And she was a very pretty goat.

He gave me another side eye and raised his eyebrows.

Me: I was kidding.

Him: Good. I was talking about your sexual habits with Michelle. How many times a week were you having sex before you became impotent?

Me: Do you have to use that word?

Him: I can use ED, but it's essentially the same thing.

Me: Let's use ED. It sounds less... emasculating.

Him: Very well. Before your ED problem surfaced, how many times a week did you have intercourse?

Me: You mean with Michelle or with the goat?

Him: I'm gonna fire you as a patient.

Me: Sorry. Before I went to Europe we made love two or three times a week. While I was gone, not at all, although I noticed the mail man didn't seem too happy to see me when I returned.

Him: And did you masturbate at all while you were abroad?

He: No.

Him: You probably should have. Your body may have taken your self-imposed abstinence as a sign you were no longer interested.

Me: Yes. Looking back I wish I had.

Him: So you went from three times a week to a screeching halt. And now you want to go back to the way it was before? Two or three times a week?

Me: Yes. That would be wonderful. For me and for Michelle, and probably the goat too.

Him: Hey, stop it with the goat, will you?

Me: I'll have you know I only fuck female goats. I'm not weird or anything.

Him: Want me to send you for a psych eval?

Me: Sorry. I'll shut up now.

He said that, in his opinion, based on all my lab results and stress test and existing conditions and sexual habits, that Viagra was probably best for me.

He said that if Viagra didn't work for me, we'd try Cialis. But that there were factors which led him to believe Viagra should be my first choice.

He also told me (pay attention, this is important) that he wanted me to use Viagra only as a last resort.

Not to take it just because I was too lazy to do other things to bring on an erection.

I asked him why not.

He said that men who take ED drugs as a first line of defense can become dependent on it. In other words, they lose their ability to get hard without it. And then, if they ever have to stop using it because for medical reasons, they're out of luck. They no longer have the ability to get an erection without it. And their days of enjoying intercourse with the woman (or goat) of their choice is gone forever.

"Do whatever you can to give yourself an erection the old fashioned way. Have Michelle help. And if nothing seems to be working, take a Viagra. Either take a short break while it takes effect, or do other things for awhile that don't involve intercourse. But give the other things a chance to work first."

He prescribed me four tablets of Viagra in the 50 mg size, scheduled a follow-up a month later, and wished me good luck.

From Michelle:

I was so excited when Jacob brought home the Viagra. I envisioned our troubles as being over forever. I thought he could just pop one whenever one of us was in the mood and we'd make love until the crack of dawn.

Then he explained Paul's stipulations. That we only use it after we've tried other means of getting him hard.

Still, it sounded reasonable.

We made love that night because both of us were looking forward to trying out our new miracle drug.

But we didn't need it that night. Jacob was able to get hard fairly easily. He said he supposed it was because he'd thought of making love to me pretty much nonstop since he left Paul's office and "willed himself" into it.

Two or three days later we get frisky again with different results. Try as I might, I just couldn't coax his little soldier into standing at attention.

So he very happily popped the magic pill and we went on to other things.

About forty minutes later he was hard. I mean, rock hard, and we enjoyed an extremely pleasurable and extended session of intercourse.

He never softened at all until he came. Never waivered. He was just as hard when he came as when he first inserted himself into me.

It was, in a word, wonderful.

From Jacob:

The Viagra worked great the first night we had to use it. And it's continued to work great every time we've used it since then.

A couple more things about it… Paul told me when I went back for my follow-up that Viagra, like any medication, can lose its potency over time. That if I took it exclusively three times a week for several years, it might not work for me as well after three years as it did for the beginning.

That was another reason he's hesitant to prescribe it as the first line of defense against erectile dysfunction.

"It's fine to use an ED medication as a crutch. Or as a backup. But if it's your first solution every time, your body might forget that manual stimulation or

other means are even options. And if you ever have to go back to those means, you may well find they no longer work."

At my follow-up, Paul prescribed four tablets, this time for the larger one milligram size.

Him: Now I'm not going to put this on the bottle, but when you get this prescription filled I want you to use a pill cutter and cut each of them in half. And only take half a tablet each time. Take it only when you need it, and never two nights in a row.

Me: Um... okay. But why not just give me the smaller size?

Him: Because Viagra is an expensive drug. And your insurance is cheap. They'll only approve four tablets per month regardless of the tablet's size. This way you'll have eight doses per month instead of four.

Me: What will happen if I forget your instructions and take a full tablet? Will my dick get harder?

Him: No. You'll just run out of pills faster.

Me: And why can't I have sex two nights in a row if I want?

Him: I never said you couldn't have sex two nights in a row. I just said I didn't want you to take Viagra two nights in a row. As with any prescription medication, you want to take the least amount possible to get the desired affect. With a lot of men, the effects of Viagra will linger for more than a day. If you use it one night, and manual stimulation or other means to get an erection the second night, there may well be enough residual Viagra left in your system to give you a boost for the second night as well.

Me: Wow! It works for two nights?

Him: In some men, yes.

A friend of mine who has a battle-related war injury and is treated by the Veteran's Administration told me the other day told me they have the same policy. They'll only prescribe four tablets of Viagra per month.

I think it's a damn shame that anyone, much less an insurance company, presumes they have the right to tell us how many times we can have sex with our wife each month. You can damn sure bet those insurance company fat cats approve as many tablets as they want for their own use.

If you're on a budget and on good terms with your doctor, and if he says 50 MG are enough for you, see if he'll consider prescribing the larger size instead. Promise you'll cut them in half and take half a tablet only when you need to.

But explain to him that keeping Mama happy requires intercourse more than four times a month.

Hopefully he'll understand.

Erectile Dysfunction Tool Box Thus Far: 12 Items

1. Frequent penis stimulation
2. Pin stimulation to penis head
3. Eat well. Diet is everything
4. Enlist your doctor's help
5. A good selection of written erotica
6. Play. Experiment. Find new things to love
7. Water is our friend. Drink lots of it.
8. Limit caffeine
9. Ice can be nice
10. Try warming oils as a stimulant
11. Porn as a visual mood setter
12. ED Medications as a backup, not as a go-to

Chapter 11: *Get in the habit of holding some back*

Not every man can do this, but it's well worth the effort to try

Okay, this little trick won't work for all men. But it'll work for a lot of you.

And granted, it takes some effort and some practice.

But if you can master the technique, it'll help you tremendously in achieving an erection next time you need one.

What we're talking about here is limiting the amount of ejaculate you release when you have your orgasm.

Many of you are saying, "What? I have a choice?"

The short answer is… maybe.

Some men (our Jacob included) have the ability, under the right circumstances, to stop the flow early, before their testicles are completely emptied.

To understand this, let's look at the whole purpose of the testicles.

They are for making, and storing, semen. That's it. That's the only reason they exist. To make sure that when it comes time to make a baby they have the stuff ready and available to allow the man to do his part.

And you thought they were also meant to be a target for angry girlfriends to kick. No, not at all. That's just a fringe benefit. For her, not for you.

Most people think the entire load of ejaculate, or semen, is made up of sperm.

The fact is, sperm makes up only a tiny part of the semen. Most of it is just a delivery vehicle to get the sperm into the female's body and to the eggs it's meant to fertilize.

Okay. That's what the balls are for. But they, by themselves, have no way to enable the man who hauls them around all day to deposit his load into the prospective mother of his choice.

That's where the penis comes in. Obviously the sperm delivery systems that are the testicles does no good without a penis to facilitate the whole delivery process.

In that regard, the penis and testicles work together to plant the fertilizer of life onto (or in close proximity) to the seed of life.

Still with us?

Good.

But they themselves can't make the man find the woman he needs to further the species.

Nor can they encourage the woman of his choice to play ball. After all, sex is messy.

That's where the brain comes in to help bring everything together.

The brain is in charge of something we call "attraction." It makes the woman attractive so that he wants to deposit his load into her.

It makes the man attractive to the woman so she's willing to allow him to deposit it there.

And the brain recognized the whole "reward" thing. To sweeten the pot, it gives us orgasms as rewards for our efforts to further the species.

And that, boys and girls, is a nutshell (and way oversimplistic) explanation of how procreation works.

Of course, there are many more things at play here.

The capacity of testicles is not finite.

They can only hold so much semen.

When they start to get full, men tend to become more apt to look around for a sex partner. Or is more likely to make advances on his wife or girlfriend.

The testicles pretty much work nonstop, twenty four hours a day, to produce that sperm and the semen it's mixed with. It wants the man to be ready to deliver the sperm anytime.

However, when they get full or close to full, the pressure starts to build. The result is a crude term men often refer to as "blue balls."

"Blue balls" are sensitive to the touch, and can make it uncomfortable for men to walk or sit, or pretty much anything else.

When a man uses another rather crude term, and says he's "horny," he likely has a case of blue balls, or is close to it.

Just how long it takes for a man to develop blue balls after his last sex session varies on several things. The man's physical makeup, his testosterone level, his sexual appetite in general, how often he has sex, the availability of willing sexual partners, among others.

Here's the thing. Whether a man's testicles are full or close to full affects his ability to get an erection.

And that makes sense if you think about it. If the testicles are full of semen that wants and needs to get out, it's only natural for the brain to help facilitate the whole sex process.

And the first step in facilitating the sex process, at least for the man, is to get an erection.

They're all tied together, you see, in an intricate orchestration meant to empty the testicles and allow them to start producing more.

That's when the brain steps in and says, "I'm gonna make you feel horny, dude, so you start looking for a place to shoot that stuff."

That's also why you guys lose all interest in sex the moment you ejaculate. Because your testicles are empty. The pressure is all gone.

Here's the question we set out to answer:

What if it didn't have to be all or nothing? What if we could train ourselves not to empty our testicles completely, but to leave some of the semen behind?

It stands to reason that if some were left behind, they would fill up again faster, the brain would send that horniness fairy sooner, and we'd be able to get another erection sooner.

Like maybe in a couple of days instead of a week or more.

Makes sense, doesn't it?

It's just too darn bad it's impossible to do that.

Only shoot half a load, we mean, and save the rest for another day.

Isn't it?

Impossible?

Maybe not.

In fact, definitely not.

Some Indians have been practicing the technique for generations. We're talking about men who live in India, not Native Americans.

It's doable for most (but not all) men. For most men, it merely takes practice.

From Jacob:

I'll admit, this technique has been the hardest one for me to master. I think it's partly because I tend to lose my mind when I have an orgasm. I'm lost in the moment, and the last thing I want to think about is, "Hey, I need to save some so I have an easier time getting an erection next time."

I have a bad habit of frequently saying instead, "Oh, to hell with it. This feels too good to stop."

It's also because, even when my head is in the right place and I'm able to pull up short, there's such a small window to hit. And if you don't hit that window, your body takes over and you can no longer control it.

It just happens on its own, the way nature intended. I empty my testicles and then they have to start all over again to fill the empty space.

Oh, don't let me mislead you. I have had limited success at this technique. Just not as much as I'd like to have had. And I'm still working to get batter at it.

And it really is effective in shortening the recovery time, and making it easier to get an erection a couple of days later. It makes sense. The fuller the testicles, the more the semen is going to want out. And the hornier our brain makes us feel.

As I see it, those are the two biggest difficulties with this technique:

- Keeping your mind on the goal, when all your body wants to do is give you an orgasm

- Hitting that window, between the time your orgasm starts and the split second you have to stop it.

The articles we read made it sound so simple: As the first flush of pleasure hits your brain, simply turn off the spigot. That first rush that tells you your orgasm is starting, you have to stop. Completely and immediately. Just slam the brakes on and come to a complete and total stop.

I know. It's not easy. Believe me, I know from experience.

But if you can train yourself to do that, two things will happen.

You'll still have your orgasm. Granted, it won't be as powerful or as prolonged. But you'll still have one.

You'll likely be a bit disappointed at first. After all, it'll go against everything you've ever wanted to achieve sexually. You may even pout like a little boy whose mother took his candy away from him.

But if you look at it another way, that this will help you get another orgasm two, three, four nights in the future (and another chance to have an orgasm), it's a little easier to handle.

After all, two orgasms are better than one. There's no denying that fact.

The second thing that'll happen when coming to a complete stop is that you will ejaculate. That much is inevitable.

But... you won't ejaculate your whole load. Much of it will be left behind.

And that, my friends, is the whole purpose of this particular exercise.

Michelle asked me a couple of weeks ago what I meant about having to "hit the window."

I thought about it a bit, trying to put it into terms she could understand.

"Picture yourself standing aside a roadway with a baseball in your hand. And a car is coming by at seventy miles an hour. Its back window is rolled down, and your job is to throw that ball into that window."

She asked, "And the car is going seventy miles an hour?"

I said, "Yes."

She said, "That's pretty hard."

I said, "Now you understand."

Then she said something that sounded absolutely ludicrous at the time, but which turned out to be very profound.

She said, "Why not slow the car down to, say, thirty miles an hour?"

From Michelle:

He looked at me as though I'd grown a second set of ears or something.

He said, "What do you mean?"

I told him he always picked up his pace tremendously when he felt he was getting ready to cum. He's been that way in all the years we've been making love. But apparently he never realized it before.

He was incredulous. He said, "Do I really?"

I told him he sped up with all the subtlety of a caveman dragging his woman by the hair.

I said, "Why not just slow down? You know it'll happen. It always does. You'll still have your orgasm. You'll still cum, but maybe by going slower it'll be easier for you to hit your window."

So he did. He tried it. And it turned out we both liked it.

I always enjoyed, as we made love, when he increased his speed. It was very passionate for both of us. It always told me he was getting close, and was my cue to verbally encourage him. And, as he entered his first throes of orgasm, to hold him close to me. To pull him as far inside of me as I could.

It's always been that way.

So this whole 'holding back' thing... it was something new that both of us had to learn.

Now, we both enjoy it better. "It" being intercourse, of course.

I suspect that at least part of it is just because it's a new experience for us. It's brought something new into our sex life that had gotten a bit humdrum over the years.

Don't tell Jacob I said that.

Oh, we're still having intercourse the same way. Still using our same favorite positions.

But we're doing it at a slower pace than before. Making it easier for him to throw that baseball through that car window.

And I'm not leaving it up to him. I'm in it with him. It's that whole "teamwork" thing. We saw his ED as a battle we both needed to fight together. We've been standing side by side throughout this fight, and this was just another fight we needed to face... together.

The articles we read said the only time he could experience his orgasm, yet still be able to hold back most of his cum, was at what they called "first flush."

Not flush as in a reddened face. But rather the first flush of pleasure he felt when his orgasm began.

I said, "I can help you with that."

He asked, "How? You can't feel it."

I told him I didn't have to feel it. I could see it. For years I could always tell when his orgasm was starting. For at the exact moment he feels that "first flush" his face starts to contort. For lack of a better description, he winces at that point.

Again, we were in it together.

We resolved to work on two things once we delved into this.

The first was to regulate his pace. To make sure he doesn't speed up when he feels he's getting close.

I have to admit, this part was a little bit hard for me, too. I'd always enjoyed the way he "rode me hard," as he put it, while he was having his orgasm. There was a wild abandonment in the way he did it, an unbridled passion.

But going slower from start to finish was nice in its own way.

The second thing we've worked on is my coming to a dead stop as soon as his face begins to wince.

This was a bit hard for me as well. I used to love to "call him home," so to speak. Before, when I sensed he was starting his orgasm, I was very vocal in my encouragement.

"Come on, baby, let me have it. I want every drop." Or, even more graphically, "Fuck me hard, baby. Don't stop."

To be honest, I missed that a little. So did he.

But we both agree it's worth the change for a couple of reasons.

First of all, he's not always successful in saving some of his load, but when he is, we know we'll be rewarded.

Rewarded by his having a much easier time getting hard the next time we make love a day or two or three later. For even after his orgasm, his testicles are still half full.

Secondly, by not emptying his balls completely, he doesn't get as sensitive as he does when he drains them dry. He also doesn't go flaccid as quickly.

And that's nice in its own way. Because after we stop and let his orgasm run its course, he can begin stroking again, and we can continue intercourse (albeit at a slower place) for several more minutes.

And that's really really cool.

From Jacob:

The technique is simple, really.

Michelle watches my face and feels my body's movement while we have intercourse. When she feels me speeding up, as I have a bad habit of doing when I'm nearing the end, she'll squeeze my hips with her hands and remind me not to.

She's not demanding about it.

She merely reminds me, "a little slower, baby," or "not so fast, baby."

The other thing she does is come to a dead stop as soon as she sees me make that face that tells her I'm getting ready to ejaculate.

She calls it my "o-face." The o stands for orgasm. I think she got that from a movie.

Anyway, once we get me hard using whichever tool or tools happens to be working on that particular night, we make love just as we always did, albeit it at a slower and more consistent pace.

When I feel the "first flush" of my orgasm, I stop and wait for it to pass. At the same time she stops moving, to lessen the friction between her vagina and my penis.

Also at the same time, I try very hard to stop ejaculating.

At first, I'll admit, stopping my ejaculation was darn near impossible. I suspect you'll feel the same way.

But if you stick with it, you'll get better with practice.

When we started this process Michelle said we needed a baseline. A goal to shoot for.

She asked me to masturbate in front of her. She counted the number of times I squirted (rather crude, but probably the term we're all most familiar with).

Anyway, I squirted seven times.

Our goal was to cut that in half, which (in our best estimate) would leave maybe a third of my semen in my testicles for use at another time.

After six months, I'm now able to stop most times after the second squirt, although it does tend to dribble a little.

This is provided I don't miss the window. If I go one or two strokes past the window, it's too late. I've lost control and ejaculate everything.

So even after you master this technique, it's still a constant battle.

From Michelle:

The results of this technique is its own reward. Once your men are able to control their ejaculations, they can leave some behind and make it easier to get an erection the next time.

*And... at least in our case, our lovemaking is slower and (I think) more sensuous than before. And those few short minutes he can still make love to me **after** he cums (which he couldn't do before) make this worth the effort.*

Remember... not all men are able to master this technique. But for those of you who can, it's worth the time and trouble you go through to get there.

Chapter 12:   *Experiment with different sexual positions.*

Get away from the vanilla of the missionary style and to something more suitable for your needs

We researched this topic extensively because, well, we're always looking for new ways to spice up our sex lives.

We've always done that, even before the ED monster reared its very ugly head.

And that includes experimenting with different sex positions.

We read a study that said most married couples have only two or three sexual positions on their bedtime menu.

We only have two or three favorites, but we have many more that we've tried and enjoyed, and which we may pull out of our bag and try on any given night.

Since we declared war on ED, though, we've been using certain positions more and more.

Basically (but not exclusively) those positions which facilitate access to Jacob's penis and testicles.

Consider it logically, and it makes a lot of sense.

One of the key tools you use to make your man hard is physical stimulation. Massaging his penis and testicles.

So why stop, just because he's hard and you're making love?

Good question. Thanks for asking.

Many men don't have so much a problem getting hard as staying that way. And it stands to reason that stimulation during intercourse might be able to help.

After all, if it was your wife playing with your penis and testicles which made you hard to begin with, wouldn't it make sense that if she continued to do so you'll stay that way?

At least it sounds good in theory.

The trouble is, as those of us who suffer from ED know all too well, not all theories pan out.

And, frustrating as it is, some work one day but not the next.

Still, this is a method of kicking the ED monster's butt that seems to help us. Our thinking is that it can help some of you too, if you're willing to apply it.

From Michelle:

One of the things Jacob and I decided to do when we started this project was to talk to as many of our friends as possible.

We did so openly and without pretense. We were up front with our friends, and told them about our project. We told them that anything they told us might wind up in the book, but that we would tell them ahead of time if we were using their words and experiences. We also assured them we would use pseudonyms if they wanted us to, or only their real first names if that was their preference.

We found out early on that men for the most part do not want to discuss their ED problems with their friends.

We're not sure why, exactly. We think it's a pride thing. And that maybe they're embarrassed. But a man who's perfectly willing and ready to tell his male friends he's having prostate problems and has to get up to pee four times a night, or to tell of his heart problems or his diabetes or his bad knees, won't utter a word about his ED. Not even if sharing ideas with his friends might help him.

It boggles the mind.

I got many times the information Jacob got by talking to the wives and girlfriends.

The other thing I learned during the process was that ED doesn't just happen to older people.

We have good friends I'll call Sally and Jim. They're in their thirties.

And they too suffer with occasional bouts of ED. I asked Sally how often.

She said three or four times a month.

I said to count her lucky stars. That we have to deal with it all the time.

She countered by saying her mother in law confided to her that's the way Jim's father started out. And then, in his early forties, he went limp and stayed that way.

Jim's parents did what generations of people suffering from ED have always done. They just learned to live without sex.

But Sally and Jim don't want to live without sex. They're very interested in this project and have already adapted some of the techniques which are helping us.

One of the things I've queried all my friends about is the sexual positions they use.

A surprising number never deviate from the traditional man-on-top, face to face, so called "missionary" position.

And normally there's nothing wrong with that. It's tried and true, and has worked to produce many an orgasm for both parties involved, probably since the beginning of mankind.

Not to mention a lot of babies.

The problem is two-fold, at least from the standpoint of couples suffering from ED.

First of all, it's boring. Especially if you do it every single time you make love.

And second, it doesn't allow the wife the freedom to massage her lover's balls, or his cock, during sex. Not at all. Sure, you wouldn't think he'd need the added encouragement once he's penetrated you.

But sadly, that's not necessarily the case. For some men, penetration isn't enough. As good as it feels for him inside of you, sometimes he needs more.

Alas, that's why getting hard is only half the battle. Staying hard is the other half.

Okay, let's tackle these in order.

We'll go with my contention that the missionary position is boring. You may or may not agree, but I'll explain my logic, and we'll deal with that first.

Do you like Coca Cola?

I do. I like it a lot. It's my soft drink of choice. And other than the two cups of coffee I drink first thing in the morning to bring me out of my zombie state, it's probably my favorite thing to drink each day.

But I don't drink Coca Cola exclusively.

I don't drink it first thing in the morning, and then again all day long every single time I'm thirsty.

Wanna know why?

Because as good as it is, and as much as I like it, I'd get sick of it if that was all I drank.

That's why.

So why are we talking about Coca Cola in a book about ED?

Because we can get tired of anything, no matter how much we love it, if that's all we have.

Jacob tells me there's no better feeling in the world than when he first slides his penis into my eagerly waiting vagina. He says the first few thrusts always make him feel as though he's died and gone to heaven.

I can definitely relate, for I feel the same way.

He asked me when the ED monster first strolled into our bedroom and roared at us how I'd feel I we had to give up intercourse completely. I told him my feelings for him wouldn't change in the slightest. I'd still love him as much as I ever did. But that I'd be lying if I said I wouldn't miss it. Intercourse is the single most intimate way a couple can bond. Everything else is nice. But intercourse is the gravy on the potatoes. The cherry on the banana split. The one thing a couple can share that no one else can share in.

I didn't want to give it up. Neither did he. That's why he played the role of my hero once again. He reached up and punched that ED monster and said it wasn't going to win.

That we were going to find a way to defeat it.

Actually we found lots of ways, each which worked for us in varying degrees. That's where our concept of building a "toolbox" came from.

One of the biggest tools in our toolbox was changing the way we made love.

We still do the missionary position sometimes. We both still like it because we can hold each other and kiss while we're making love.

But missionary is no longer our go-to position. It may be one of three or four positions we try on any given night.

We bought one of those hokey books on sexual positions on the internet, with the intention of trying every single one of them.

That quickly went out the window when we discovered most of them couldn't be done unless you're both rail thin and in your early twenties, and have the flexibility of a professional gymnast.

We were none of the above.

So we discarded most of the positions in the book and looked for a few which fit our particular needs.

Our needs, as we saw them, were positions which allowed me to reach his dick and balls with either my hands or my mouth.

In that manner, whatever else we happened to be doing at the time I could continue to stimulate him.

Jacob loves giving me oral sex. He says that it's his second favorite part of our lovemaking sessions, just behind penetration.

And I have to admit, I like it too. A lot. A WHOLE LOT.

The problem was it was hard to incorporate it into our lovemaking session. If we started out with him going down on me, he always went soft while he was doing it. Then, when I was hot and bothered and begging him to put himself into me, we had to stop and make him hard again first.

Our solution was to switch to what we all know as the "sixty nine" position, or to the "modified sixty nine position."

I think most of you know which ones I'm talking about, but will explain briefly for those who don't.

In the traditional sixty nine position, one of you lies on his or her back and the other lies on top, facing in the opposite direction. Doing so gives one's face access to the other's genitals and allows the couple to perform oral sex at the same time.

The modified sixty nine calls for the couple to lie next to each other, both on their right side and facing each other. Same effect, but with this one it's a bit harder to reach the genitals.

A couple of very important things to note: This isn't for everyone. Most of us have gained a few extra pounds as we've aged, and extra pounds can make this one more difficult.

I'm not heavy, but I'm soft. Jacob is considerably lighter. So he always takes the top position.

At the same time, though, he doesn't want to bear down on me and make me uncomfortable.

He avoids this by getting on his tiptoes, as though he were doing a push-up. And by resting on his elbows, atop a pillow he places on either side of me. I can still feel his weight, but it's not uncomfortable for me.

In this position, he can perform oral on me at the same time I'm performing oral on him.

The beauty of this position is that I always achieve at least one orgasm. Sometimes two or three, if I'm not too sensitive after the first one.

That's important (and not just because it feels good).

It's important because there are nights when we can't get him hard no matter what we try. And on those nights Jacob can go to sleep knowing he gave me pleasure. I've told him a zillion times there's no need to feel guilty about the whole ED thing. That it's not his fault. But he's confessed to me that despite my words he'll always feel pangs of guilt when he can't (as he puts it), "perform."

In this position he's able to perform, meaning he gives me great pleasure, in another way.

Our preferred outcome of this position, of course, is to use it as a prelude to intercourse.

Even after all these years, I still find it incredibly sexy to have him towering over me, his cock hanging down and eagerly waiting for me to take it into my mouth. I still love sucking on him almost as much as he does.

From Jacob:

Another position we've had great success with is the modified doggy position.

We've tried the doggy position, which calls for both of us to stand on the bedroom floor, and for Michelle to bend forward and place her hands on her knees. I then hold her by the hips and enter her vagina from behind.

We didn't like that position because putting her head down for several minutes made Michelle light-headed.

The modified doggy position, however, worked much better for us.

With this position Michelle still has her feet on the floor, but the top half of her body lies across the bed.

The only bad thing about this position is that I no longer have the option of cupping or fondling her breasts while we make love.

But she can easily reach back and cup or gently massage my testicles, which helps prevent me from going soft during intercourse.

Which is the whole point of our experimenting with various positions to begin with.

If you try this position and it works for you, it might require some modifications to your bed.

Our bed is rather high to begin with. It was just the right height for Michelle to stand next to it with both feet on the floor and then lay her body across it.

I'm four inches taller than Michelle. That's not a great amount, and we found that by spreading my feet slightly wider than my shoulders I could still maintain a firm footing while lowering my body so my penis lined up with her vagina.

If your bed is too low, and if you expect to use this position often, you might consider bed risers.

They're simple blocks that go under your bed's legs or wheels and raise them up six or eight inches. The tops are recessed just a bit to prevent the legs or wheels from falling off of them, and they're sold on the internet and at some department stores for a few dollars.

From Michelle:

The last position we've incorporated into out permanent lovemaking menu is a side position. It's a bit harder to describe, but I'll try my best to help you visualize it.

In this position I lie on my side in the center of the bed with, my bottom leg perfectly straight.

My top leg is bent at the knee.

Jacob climbs on top of me, his two legs straddling my straight lower leg, and inserts himself into me.

From this position I can easily reach his testicles. I can gently massage them, or just cup them in my hands. He says the sensation, either way, is a great turn-on for him and helps him to stay hard.

One important note about this one:

There was an article we read on the internet which suggested this as a good tool for maintaining an erection... which we certainly agree with.

However... the same article suggested that the woman squeeze her lover's testicles as an additional way of keeping him turned on.

We experimented with that method, and Jacob didn't like it at all. Remember what we said before.

Men are like snowflakes in that no two are alike. What turns one man on doesn't necessarily turn on the next guy.

And some men, like my Jacob, have very sensitive testicles.

If you experiment with squeezing them, do so carefully and gently, until you find out what constitutes pleasure and what borders on discomfort.

These are the positions which worked for us.

We tied several others and discarded them for various reasons. We couldn't do some because we just weren't flexible enough. Some seemed just plain silly, and others we just didn't have the body types for.

We'd encourage you to try at least these three to see if they work for you. If they're not a good fit, try others.

We see these as beneficial for two reasons. One we've already talked about: giving you wives better access to your man's goodies so you can continue to fondle them even while you're having intercourse.

But there's a second value as well.

Any time you can add something new to your lovemaking, it brings a little more spice and excitement into the mix.

We're sure you've learned that over the years, and it's true. That's why we (the wives) have tried everything from lingerie that's very uncomfortable to bedroom games which can seem downright stupid.

The point is, we tend to get bored in the bedroom after doing the same old things year after year.

Introducing new positions at this point may just make your lovemaking sessions more exciting for him. More of a turn-on. Especially if such positions allow his lover more access to him.

And for men with ED, it's all about the excitement. Just that one little thing you haven't discovered yet might be the thing which excites him enough to help him get and stay hard.

Erectile Dysfunction Tool Box Thus Far: 14 Items

1. Frequent penis stimulation
2. Pin stimulation to penis head
3. Eat well. Diet is everything
4. Enlist your doctor's help
5. A good selection of written erotica
6. Play. Experiment. Find new things to love
7. Water is our friend. Drink lots of it.
8. Limit caffeine
9. Ice can be nice
10. Try warming oils as a stimulant
11. Porn as a visual mood setter
12. Use ED Medications as a backup, not as a go-to
13. Learn to save some for a rainy day
14. Change the mechanics of how you make love

Chapter 13:   *Mutual Masturbation*

Stop thinking of it as dirty. Think of it as fun. And useful too.

Okay, let's continue that same line of thinking… that anything which turns you guys on can help you get and stay hard.

We've discussed the snowflake principle already: how no two men are alike. And it's very true, whether you're talking about bedroom activities or anything else.

Some men love burritos. Some hate them. Some men love golf. Others hate it. Some men love big boobs. Others prefer small ones. Still others (most, probably) don't care how big boobs are as long as they're attached to the woman they love.

There are some things which nearly all men love, although many of them won't admit it because they were raised to think they were dirty and should be done behind closed doors.

One of them is watching their woman masturbate.

Another is masturbating themselves while their woman watches.

If this is something you haven't done, it's time to ask your partner if they'd be interested in doing it. You might be surprised, when you're both honest with your feelings and desires, that the concept turns you on.

Or at least intrigues you a bit.

It's okay to be shy at first. Especially for you women.

But you've done it before, you know you have, when your husband wasn't around.

Just do it the same way again. If it helps, do it with your eyes closed so you can't see him watching you, at least until you're used to it.

And watch him. Don't watch his face or his eyes while he masturbates. Watch his penis. There's something supremely sexy about watching your man stroke his own penis. And him watching you watch him so closely will excite him too.

One thing we want to emphasize... we're not necessarily suggesting that he masturbate to ejaculation. We use this mainly as a means of turning Jacob on enough to make him hard. We usually progress from that point to intercourse.

However... not always. Sometimes our mutual masturbation sessions are such a turn-on to both of us that we both stimulate ourselves to orgasm.

And that's okay.

Because a rich and rewarding sex life doesn't always begin and end in intercourse.

A rich and regarding sex life includes a variety of sexual activities.

We're big believers in the old adage *if it feels good and doesn't hurt anybody, do it.*

From Michelle:

Early on in our relationship, so long ago it seems like forever, I asked Jacob to masturbate in front of me.

I was curious. I knew that young men of his age did such things. We were in college then, and lived in a college town. There were several adult theaters in town where men could go and rent a private "booth" to sit in where they were hidden from view for a few extra dollars.

My best friend Nancy was the receptionist for one such theater. She was strikingly beautiful, blonde and busty, which I suspect was why she got the job.

The thing she loved about the job was that it paid so well. About four times what I made waiting tables. The manager told her he paid her so well because she was "good for business." He never explained to her why, but we assumed she drew in a lot of boys because of her looks.

The thing she hated about the job was that each evening after the theater closed, she had to help the projectionist clean up. And that meant going into the theater itself, pulling back the curtains of the private "booths" and mopping the cum off the floor.

She told me the theater provided a roll of paper towels and a garbage can to collect their semen, but that some of the men didn't bother to use them.

So I knew that men of that age did that. Many, according to Nancy, came in every night she was there.

The night I asked Jacob to jerk off he looked at me like I was crazy, but then complied.

I was aroused. I don't know why. I supposed it was because I could see the pleasure on his face, even though his eyes were clamped tightly closed and I sensed he was a bit embarrassed.

After he finished he said he couldn't have intercourse for awhile. I wasn't aware of what he called the "cum and done policy" and asked what he meant. He explained that after he ejaculated he needed some recovery time. I never knew that. Boy, was I dumb back then.

Anyway, we found other pleasurable things to do while we waited, and eventually were able to have intercourse.

As we lay in the bed afterwards, I asked why it embarrassed him to jerk off in front of me. He said he didn't know. Perhaps, he thought, because it had always been such a personal and private thing to him. Something he hid. Something society considered "dirty."

I told him I didn't think it was dirty at all. I told him I thought it was sexy. The only thing I didn't particularly like about it was the recovery time he needed before we could continue.

I also told him that if it wasn't for his recovery time it would have been something I'd have liked to do frequently in our warm-up to having intercourse.

I did ask him to do it again occasionally (particularly late in my pregnancies when I lost all desire for passion but still enjoyed watching him). He eventually stopped being embarrassed and enjoyed performing for me.

One of the things we stumbled across on the internet was that mutual masturbation can be a tool for helping with ED.

It apparently doesn't work for everyone, but it works very well for some.

Jacob was out doing yard work when I found the reference and I bookmarked the page so I could share it with him.

He came in all sweaty, which I somehow found sexy when he was a young man. Now I just regard it as yuck.

I told him I found something fun on the internet that might help make his dick hard and he smiled and wanted to know what it was. I said, "No way, Bucko.

Not until you come out of the shower smelling like a newborn baby's butt."

Or at least a clean man.

After he showered we read the article and then discussed the whole topic of mutual masturbation.

It was then I realized for the first time how much he loved to jerk off for me. But not to completion. In the early days, as I said, he would occasionally do it until he ejaculated, then we'd do other things until he was able to get hard again. Back in those days (when we were in our late twenties) his erections came often, sometimes several times in a day. So letting him ejaculate wasn't that big a deal. We could still have a great sex session even after he did.

As the years went by, though, we realized how precious a commodity his ejaculate (and erections) really are. And we tried to conserve both of them as much as possible.

The solution is for him to jerk off for me sometimes, but only until he's hard enough to put himself in me. Once he's hard enough to do that, he generally stays hard enough to finish.

He told me on that day, as we perused that particular article, that he'd gotten over his embarrassment at masturbating in front of me long ago. Now it was more a turn-on for him.

At the same time, he once struggled with the whole notion. Did his fondness for being watched while spanking his monkey (or whacking his chicken, or beating his meat, or whichever silly term you want to choose) mean he was perverted in some way? Would it lead to other, more bizarre behavior? Would he turn into one of those creeps who hides in the bushes and waits for little girls to walk by so he can jump out and masturbate in front of them?

The answer, of course, is no. But he admitted to worrying about such silly things.

We pursued that line of thinking by talking to a good friend of ours, who just happens to be one of the most highly regarded clinical psychologists in the state.

He told us that the pleasure a man derives while his lover watches him masturbate is perfectly normal and not deviant at all. It's born from the knowledge that at that particular place and time, he has the undivided attention of the woman he loves and who loves him. And the one he strives so hard to please in the bedroom. And that at that particular place and time, I am being turned on by watching him. And that I want nothing more than for him to get pleasure by what he's doing, And that (here's the kicker), I derive my own pleasure by watching him jerking off.

In other words, Masturbating in front of one's lover (by women as well as men) is normal and just another option of lovemaking. He said in that regard, it's no different than oral sex or anal sex or manual stimulation by one's partner or the use of a vibrator during sex.

He said most cultures (and Americans are among the worst) are still hung up in thinking that it really isn't sex unless intercourse is involved.

And that's just not the case. If it involves a prick, or a pussy, and it feels good for one or both parties, it's sex.

Period.

Anyway, back to my point. Jacob got over his embarrassment at jerking off in front of me many years ago. Since then it's become a turn on for him. Especially when it's accompanied by my masturbating for him.

For the record, I never had a problem doing it in front of him. I'd always enjoyed touching myself, even as an adolescent. I've always been very outgoing. Jacob calls me "The life of every party and most PTA meetings." I've called him "My old stick in the mud."

Lovingly, of course.

That's one key difference between us. I make a point to talk to everyone at a party. That's actually my goal when we socialize. To meet everyone there and get to know them a little. Jacob, on the other hand, tends to seek out his good friends and hang around with them for most of the night.

Whether it's that tendency that made him embarrassed to masturbate in front of me in our younger days, while I pretty much spread my legs wide and said, "Hey, Sailor, lookie what I've got. Wanna watch me touch it?" had anything to do with those personal traits, I can't say.

But the fact was, it never bothered me to masturbate for him. Not even the first time. It still doesn't. In fact, I rather enjoy it. It makes me feel that after all these years, he still finds pleasure in looking at my naked body.

Masturbation on his part can be a tremendous asset in helping make his ED manageable. Encourage him to do it in front of you. And while he's doing it, tell him how you admire it. Compliment him. Tell him how attractive he is. How lucky you are to have him. How much you enjoy making love to him.

Don't be afraid to talk dirty to him. Most men like it. Tell him there's no better feeling in the world than when he slides his hard cock into you.

Offer to help him by gently massaging his balls, and running your fingertips very softly up and down his upper thighs (one of a man's erogenous zones).

And if he wants you to, masturbate for him too.

Then, when that dick gets hard, pounce on it!

From Jacob:

Michelle asked me awhile back why men like it when they talk dirty. She asked if it went back to a man's caveman days, when sex was just a raw act of passion, devoid of feelings or compassion or mutual pleasure.

I said no, it's because men are dogs.

It's a very primal instinct. A man wants to know that he is desired. When he's in the mood for sex and his wife rolls over half-heartedly and says, "Okay, but try not to muss my hair," it does nothing to boost his self-esteem and reinforce the (perhaps false) belief that he is a devastatingly handsome sexual dynamo.

When she says, "Oh, baby, get that big beautiful cock hard and put it in me, then pound me hard until we both cum a hundred times," there is no doubt. He's better than Superman, Batman and Captain America all rolled into one.

That's a rather simplistic example, but for many (maybe most) men, a few choice dirty words from their woman can make them feel virile and desired.

And that can go a very long way in helping him obtain an erection.

When I masturbate for Michelle I typically use a warming lubricant and stand along the bedside. She'll typically lie on the bed in front of me and masturbate with one hand, while tenderly caressing my leg or testicles with the other.

Sometimes she'll close her eyes and moan, which is a tremendous turn-on to me and always has been. Her face flushes and her body convulses when she has an orgasm, and that's even more of a turn on.

Sometimes she'll open her eyes and prop herself up on one elbow and use the other hand to masturbate. When she does that, she positions herself so that her face is mere inches from my penis.

She won't look at my face at all. She'll study my penis as I'm stroking it, as though trying to memorize every part of it.

And that too, is a tremendous turn on. It reinforces the fact that she desires it... no, she wants it. Badly.

Sometimes she'll throw in some very descriptive verbal foreplay as a bonus: "You've got a beautiful cock, baby. I can't wait to feel that big monster sliding in and out of me... in and out..."

The entire time this is going on, of course, I'm watching her watch me. I'm watching her pleasure herself. I'm listening to her words. I'm watching her face flush and her body convulse. I'm feeling her fingertips on places I like to feel them.

And all of that together creates a very sensuous environment. One that is frequently conducive to obtaining an erection. Very frequently, in our case.

And always, one of two things happens.

Either all of that together, coaxes my penis to get erect, and I crawl onto the bed with Michelle and put myself into her and we make love the way we once did before the ED monster came along.

Or it doesn't work and we try something else in our toolbox instead.

If the former happens, we've discovered two things that help the situation tremendously. First, if I get an erection, we don't have to mess with lubricants. Michelle is plenty wet already from playing with herself. And I'm plenty lubed up from using the warming oil. So it's just a matter of climbing into the bed and slipping it in.

That's important because, as you've already found out, getting the erection is only half the battle. Keeping it is the other half. And getting an erection, only to have to stop long enough to lubricate it, is almost a guarantee it'll start to get soft again.

The other thing we noticed is that, using this method of arousal, I almost never go soft once I'm inside of her. With some of the other methods we use, I have to get moving and keep moving once my penis is in her. If I stop stroking for even a moment to catch my breath, I begin to soften.

With this particular method, using mutual masturbation as foreplay, that's not usually the case. Once I slip myself inside of her I'll typically stay hard until she has another orgasm. She'll let me know when she's close and I'll try to time mine to match hers.

Exactly why that is, I don't know. I suppose it has to do with me watching her in rapt anticipation of knowing what's coming (no pun intended). While I'm masturbating I'm very intently watching every move her body makes...

Every sound she makes.

Watching her masturbate, or watching her watch me while I masturbate, is very stimulating.

Which is, of course, the whole purpose.

From Michelle:

I think what I like most about watching him masturbate is that the closer I put my face to his cock the more excited he gets. I literally put my face inches from it. Close enough to smell its musky smell. Close enough to see the moisture leak out of the tip. Close enough to catch it in my mouth. Although I've never developed a taste for the stuff I have caught it and swallowed it a few times. That's a personal choice between you and your man.

From Jacob:

There's only one drawback about this, and depending on how you define "having sex," you may not consider it a drawback at all. If that makes no sense, allow me to explain.

Many people view the word "sex" as being interchangeable with the word "intercourse." The whole purpose of getting an erection is to have intercourse, and that's how they always end their night of lovemaking.

If that describes you and your partner, then mutual masturbation might not be for you. More on that in a minute.

Many other couples, like Michelle and I, define sex in a different way. Pretty much anything involving our genitals that feels good and results in at least one of us (hopefully both) having at least one orgasm (hopefully several) to us… counts as sex.

In other words, we don't necessarily have to have intercourse to be fulfilled. We can do lots of other stuff instead.

So, for us, obtaining an erection isn't necessarily just so I can put it inside her, although I frequently do. Sometimes I get an erection so she can jerk me off, or suck me off, or so I can jerk off in front of her.

If you are a couple which always ends the night with intercourse, this method might not be appropriate for you and here's why…

Remember a few pages back we discussed learning how to hold some back? Not to ejaculate fully, but rather to leave some semen in your testicles for the next time?

I'd like for all you guys to try to master that technique. Even if you can't master it, but can learn to do it to some degree will help with your ED issue.

The problem is, it's extremely difficult to hit that tiny window and stop short your ejaculate when you're masturbating.

No, I don't know why.

When I ejaculate during intercourse, I can stop the flow of my semen at least seven or eight out of ten times.

When I masturbate it's more like two out of ten times.

You might ask why that's important. Here's why: If you masturbate for the express purpose of getting hard or staying hard, with the intention of inserting yourself into your wife's vagina as the end goal, it's easy to go "too far." You might mean to ejaculate "a little" and then to save the rest for intercourse.

But if you're like me, there's a good chance you'll ejaculate every drop of your semen and will be done for the night.

If that does happen, try not to be disappointed. After all, you and your wife have just shared something very intimate together. And while it might not have been what you expected, you can still take the time to pleasure her in any number of ways, and then try the intercourse thing another night.

First, though, you have to get over the stigma that many people have about masturbation.

This is the 21st century. We have lots of cool things now, like electricity and vehicles that move without the aid of horses. We've been to the moon.

And not only do women have the right to vote, they're able to do any damn thing a man can do.

Yet many of us are still stuck in the mindset of the 19th century when it comes to masturbation.

It's okay. Seriously.

Get over it.

Erectile Dysfunction Tool Box Thus Far: 15 Items

1. Frequent penis stimulation
2. Pin stimulation to penis head
3. Eat well. Diet is everything
4. Enlist your doctor's help
5. A good selection of written erotica
6. Play. Experiment. Find new things to love
7. Water is our friend. Drink lots of it.
8. Limit caffeine
9. Ice can be nice
10. Try warming oils as a stimulant
11. Porn as a visual mood setter
12. ED Medications as a backup, not as a go-to
13. Learn to save some for a rainy day
14. Change the mechanics of how you make love
15. Whack your wiener for her. She'll enjoy it and it'll help with the ED

Chapter 14:   *Step on a Scale, Guys*

Losing a few extra pounds can make a huge difference

Okay, guys, let's be honest here. By show of hands, how many of you have picked up a few extra pounds as you got older?

Yeah, we thought so.

From Jacob:

Paul, my doctor, is one of those freakishly weird people who can eat anything he wants and not gain an ounce.

I hate him. I want to beat him over the head with a 1966 Chevy Impala. I probably would, but I can't lift it. Paul should be banished from the earth along with the other genetic freakazoids like him and forced to live out their days on the moon. Maybe green cheese will be the one thing which finally makes him fat.

Actually, I'm kidding. I don't hate Paul at all. He's a very good friend.

If anything, I'm jealous of Paul, because I always wanted to be one of those guys.

Me, if I'm walking down the street and pass a Dunkin' Donuts, I have to hold my breath. Because if I inhale and catch the mere scent of a glazed donut, the button pops off my pants and my waist size miraculously increases two sizes.

Michelle and I frequent an outstanding Italian restaurant called Orlando's. Paul and his wife Linda are frequently our dinner guests because Paul, although he's a successful doctor and owns a yacht and not one, but two classic BMWs, is at heart a cheapskate.

He knows I love Orlando's and will go there at the drop of a hat, and he knows I usually pick up the tab. So he suggests it often.

Also, I think he enjoys torturing me.

He knows that I'll order a half portion of cannelloni, and will force myself to eat a salad before I can touch my entrée. He knows that I will look at the basket full of garlic bread spears and will drool to the point a long line of saliva runs nonstop into my lap and soaks my trousers. But I won't partake of it.

Meanwhile, he'll order the all-you-can-eat pasta extravaganza and will get plate after plate of the stuff.

He's a sadist.

That's why he must leave this earth and go straight to the fiery pits of hell.

Paul is one of those guys who hit the genetic lottery. He can eat whatever he wants, as much as he wants, and he doesn't gain weight. Further, he's relatively healthy.

I'm not that way. I have to watch what I eat, because if I didn't I'd blow up like the Goodyear blimp.

The only solace I have is knowing I'm not alone.

There are vastly more men of my age who are like me than are like Paul.

Odds are, many of you are like me as well.

It's not our fault. That's not what I'm implying at all.

It's partly genetics, and partly just a sad side effect of aging.

And I don't have to lecture you about it, because that's your doctor's job.

Paul has the lines memorized. I know, because he says it exactly the same way every single time I go in for my physical.

   Paul: I want you to lose another fifteen pounds.
   Me: Screw you.
   Paul: I'm serious. Fifteen more pounds.
   Me: I'm serious too. Screw you.
   Paul: It'll give you more energy.
   Me: I don't need any more energy. I write for a living. I sit at my keyboard. How much energy do I need to work a keyboard?
   Paul: You'll be able to wear all those clothes in your closet that got too tight but you couldn't bring yourself to throw out. Just think of it. You can once again wear that lime green leisure suit you kept from the 1970s.
   Me: The one I wore to your first wedding?
   Paul: I think it was my fourth wedding, but yes.
   Me: Screw the old clothes. I need new ones anyway.
   Paul: If you lose fifteen pounds you'll live longer.
   Me: Living longer is way overrated.
   Paul: It may help with your erectile dysfunction.
   Me: (silent)
   Then, Me: Okay, you slimy bastard. You've got my attention. Tell me more.

It turns out that shedding just a few pounds can dramatically reduce your erection problems. I don't know how, and Paul himself couldn't say for sure. He said studies have been performed all over the world that indicate men who already have ED have fewer problems as they shed excess weight. He says nobody is quite sure why. But that it's not surprising.

After all, studies have also shown that when you shed those few extra pounds you can help yourself in a lot of different ways.

Diabetics find it easier to control their blood sugar level.

People with heart issues have fewer heart issues.

We have more energy. It's suddenly easier to go for those evening walks we've been putting off for years.

We're less stressed.

Which, by the way, we're going to discuss in a minute.

So losing a few pounds is kind of a no-brainer. The fact most of us haven't done it isn't because we don't know we should do it and need to do it.

It's because it's damn hard.

After all, those pounds go on a heck of a lot easier than they come off, am I right? Can I get an amen, brother?

Doctors have what they call an "ideal weight." Your doc can tell you what yours is. It's based on your height. That's how, no matter how much you suck in your gut at physical time, he knows instantly whether you've been following his advice to lose a few pounds or whether you've been giving into your urge to have an extra slice of pizza.

My ideal weight is 194 pounds. I haven't weighed 194 pounds since college.

But at least knowing my ideal weight gives me a goal to shoot for, even if I know I'll never achieve it.

I weighed myself this morning. I weigh 204. Ten pounds overweight, according to Paul's "Magical Chart of Sadistic Body Weight Standards."

I've been trying to get to 194 for awhile now. Michelle tells me I should just stop, be happy I've made it to 204 (I once weighed 244) and maintain it at 204.

"It's not a bad weight for you," she says. "You look better than you have in a very long time."

Deep down I know she's right. I look damn good. I feel better after losing those forty pounds, my blood sugar numbers look better and I feel more virile. And my penis does indeed get harder.

But I want to lose those last ten pounds so I can shut Paul the hell up. Just once, I'd like to go into my physical without giving the bastard the pleasure of saying those words:

"You still need to lose a few more pounds."

By the way, I'm going to kidnap Paul later and tie him up, then drive him to the Grand Canyon and throw him in. Any of you guys want to help?

From Michelle:

Jacob asked me to finish this chapter because he said he was starting to lecture you guys. He said he was starting to sound like Paul. And that's not the intent of this book. The intent of this book is to help you. Not to pound something into your head that you already know.

He also wasn't going to share with you the way he lost those forty pounds.

He said dieting and weight loss are very personal things. They're different for everybody. Each of us has to find that diet that works best for us, and what helps one person lose weight might not work for others.

But I'm his wife and I've overruled him.

After all, I'm the boss of us. It's been that way since we met. He'd argue the point, but he'd be wrong.

Here's the way I feel on the matter:

We went into this project with the knowledge there are a lot of different things which contribute to ED, and a lot of (possible) solutions to help deal with it.

We also knew going in that some things worked better for some men than they did for others. And that we'd list everything we tried to help with our ED problem which worked for us to some degree.

And realistically, we felt that Paul's weight loss did indeed help with the ED problem. We'll never know to what degree, since we were also trying a lot of other methods while he was in the process of losing the weight. But it did help.

So we'd be remiss in overlooking that aspect and not talking about it. If Jacob doesn't want to discuss it further for fear of sounding like he's lecturing you, then fine. He can go watch the news.

Like I said, am the boss, so I'll talk to you about it myself.

But I won't lecture you.

The subtitle of this book is "What Worked for Us."

So I'll merely tell you how Jacob lost his forty pounds. It may or may not work for you. If it does, that's awesome and congratulations.

If it doesn't, find another method which does work for you. Lose those extra pounds if you need to. It'll help with the ED, and it'll probably help you live longer too.

So what have you got to lose?

Besides a few extra pounds, I mean.

Jacob blames his problem with weight on genetics. And to be honest, there have been some very heavy men in his family.

So the genetics thing may hold water.

But then again, the men in his family love to eat. I've seen his brothers put away three plates of pasta at a sitting. So there's that too.

Anyway, here's what worked for us and helped Jacob lose those stubborn pounds.

For us, it was just a matter of making a few lifestyle changes.

When he was raised, Jacob wasn't allowed to leave the table until his plate was clean. The first thing he told our kids when they had kids of their own was to not carry on that tradition.

My daughter asked "Why?"

Jacob said, "Because it'll become engrained in their psyche that food is not to be left behind. For the rest of their lives they'll make a habit of always eating everything on their plates, even if they're stuffed and don't need it."

And it's true.

I've seen him stuff himself to the gills, almost to the point of throwing up. Yet he always eats that last bite and leaves his plate squeaky clean.

Here's how we solved that…

I simply put up all of our regular sized dinner plates.

I'd have thrown them away, but we entertain dinner guests a couple of times a month. When we do, I drag out the regular dinner plates and use them to serve our guests.

On those nights, however, Jacob and I still use our dessert plates.

Yes, you read that right. We eat all our meals on dessert plates.

They're only half the size of a regular dinner plate, and therefore only hold half as much food.

When I first served them I took Jacob by surprise, as I hadn't told him beforehand about the switch.

He said, "Honey, we need a new dishwasher. The old one shrunk the dishes."

I said, "Nope. We're going to use these from now on. They hold less food so we'll eat less. And I'm in it right along with you."

He said, "How big are these plates?"

I said, "I measured them. They're eight inches long."

He said, "Hey. Me too."

I said, "I know, honey. That's the only reason I put up with your foolishness."

I have to admit there's more than a grain of truth in that.

Anyway, that was the first thing we did.

And believe it or not, it works.

Jacob was generally close to full when he finished half his larger plate anyway. He kept on eating until it was empty.

Now, he eats smaller portions from a smaller plate and is generally satisfied without feeling the need to go back for more.

The second thing we did was go into the whole diet thing together.

Just as we decided to tackle the whole ED thing as a team, we used the same united front philosophy to tackle the diet.

Our logic was sound. The quickest way for a diet to fail is for the dieter to see someone close to him eating things he can't.

And I needed to lose a few pounds myself.

Part three of our plan was to go through the cupboards and refrigerator.

And we threw away all the things we knew weren't good for us.

This one, if you try it, might be a bit tricky for you.

Jacob and I were both raised in households where there wasn't a lot of money. We always had plenty to eat, but our folks certainly weren't rich. And both of us wore hand-me-downs from our older siblings.

Our parents weren't the type who would throw away perfectly good food which they'd spent their hard-won salary to purchase.

We inherited those traits. It was very hard to resist the urge to toss the food in the garbage.

We wanted to say, "Let's just push that box of macaroni and cheese to the back of the cupboard and we'll feed it to our guests."

But we knew batter. Even if it was hidden behind healthy stuff, we'd know it was back there. And in a moment of weakness, we knew we'd dig it out and eat it.

Our solution... instead of throwing it all away, we put it into three cardboard boxes and took it down to the local food bank. And that made us feel good about helping others, while at the same time helping ourselves. Lose weight, that it.

Giving away food that we loved to eat went against our grain. But we're glad we did it. And we found, amazingly enough, that giving that crap away actually saves money in the long run.

Here's why. After we got rid of the junk food, we simply stopped buying it. Jacob knew that if he picked up a four-pack of pudding cups at the supermarket I'd take them to the food bank when he wasn't looking.

I knew that if I picked up a box of cake mix, he'd do the same.

Both of us are in the mindset now that any junk we buy is like throwing away our money.

So we no longer buy junk food.

And junk food, as you know, is very expensive.

Oh, we don't go totally without.

But now in order to have a candy bar, or a couple of cookies, we have to earn them. More on that coming...

Thing three: We exercise more.

I know what you're saying. First, you're saying I'm a flaming bitch from the fiery pits of hell for even mentioning exercise. Then you're making excuses. The gym's too far away and they look at you funny, etc.

But that's not what I'm saying.

Our version of "more exercise" is more walks, which we've always loved to do anyway.

Since our early days, Jacob and I loved to walk. We'd stroll hand in hand in the park, talking about anything and everything. How we viewed the world. Our hopes and dreams. How many children we'd have, and how those children would become presidents, ambassadors and movie stars.

Later on, after our children had grown up to be con artists, criminals and mass murderers (just kidding... maybe) we still walked. We talked about where we'd gone wrong.

Now, even though the grandkids consider us "old" we still walk, and still hold hands while we do so. And still talk about anything and everything.

That's when we decided to do this book, while on one of our walks.

Anyway, our version of more exercise was more walking.

Walking, as you probably know, is one of the safest forms of exercise for people over fifty. It's heart-friendly, meaning it exercises the heart without stressing it. It's much easier on the joints than running. It doesn't require a bicycle and therefore won't get flat tires. And it doesn't require a swimming pool, which many of us either can't afford or don't want to maintain.

All it takes is a pair of good shoes and a safe place to walk.

Also, since ED is most prevalent in men over fifty, it stands to reason that many of you reading these words are indeed over fifty.

I'd suggest that if you're not already walking every day, you start. It'll not only help you shed those few extra pounds you've been desperate to lose. It'll make you healthier at the same time.

And will probably help you live longer too.

Jacob and I walked half a mile a day even before he developed ED. So we were already in the habit.

We decided to double our walk to a mile a day (1.2 kilometers for you friends who live across the pond from us) once he seriously decided to lose those extra pounds.

We laid out two courses. One of them took us through a neighborhood park a few blocks from our home.

The other took us through our neighborhood.

Why two courses? Thanks for asking.

One reason was so that we didn't get bored walking the same route night after night. On the days when the wind isn't blowing we typically walk through the park.

Sometimes it's a bit cool at night, and if it's breezy the wind can have a bitter bite to it. On those nights we walk through the neighborhood streets.

We've been doing this for several months now, long enough to get acquainted with several neighbors we hadn't known before. We'll wave at them when we see them out and sometimes stop to talk with them.

Walking is a great way to meet the neighbors and make new friends.

We often walk in the mornings too, now. One of the most enjoyable parts of our walking in the evenings was watching the sun set. It's really beautiful where we live.. And it occurred to us that on many days, we could watch it come up instead.

I love it when we're both free to walk in the mornings. The air is crisper and cleaner and it's just more... joyous, for lack of a better term.

Last winter we were walking through our neighborhood and smelled smoke. It was coming from a house where the residents were still sleeping. We pounded on their doors and windows and woke them up, where they just made it out before their home burned to the ground.

We also called the fire department, who later said a spark from the fireplace they'd left burning through the night caught a rug on fire.

The family has since become good friends. They go on and on about how Jacob and I saved their lives. I don't know about that. I think in all likelihood they would have awakened on their own once the smoke smell was strong enough.

My point, though, is that you meet the most wonderful people when you walk through your neighborhood. And you help them too. There are at least two other couples I know of who've started walking themselves because they saw us stroll by every evening.

Another benefit of walking in the morning is a habit we've developed of stopping in at a local coffee shop. We've gotten to know the owner very well, as well as some of our local police officers.

It turns out that the early morning right around sunrise is a relatively peaceful time on the streets in our town. That's when the police officers near the end of their shifts and have a few minutes of free time to start to unwind.

The first time we stopped by the coffee shop there were four officers there talking shop about a disturbance they'd quelled that night. It was a fascinating conversation.

Although hesitant at first to share the conversation with us "civilians," they warmed up a bit when we bought them each a second cup of coffee.

Since then, whenever we see police cars in the coffee shop parking lot, we make a point to stop in for a cup. They have donuts there as well, but we never partake in them. Neither do the officers. Not because they don't like donuts, but because they don't want to be stereotyped or made fun of.

Anyway, my point is that our morning walks have also enabled us to make friends with several of our local policemen. If you don't know any, get to know them. They have our backs, protect us from bad guys, and are genuinely nice people. They deserve a pat on the back and a friendly word occasionally.

Oh, and they have the most fascinating stories to tell.

We've been told more than once by our neighbors that they love to see us stroll around the neighborhood and across the park.

For one thing, we hold hands every step of the way. We've always been hand-holders, so we never really noticed. But apparently, from what we've been told by others, a hand-holding couple is exceedingly rare these days.

We've also been known to stop walking occasionally and to dance on the sidewalk, hearing music only we can hear. Some of the neighbors have come to know us as the "dancing couple," we've heard. Of course, I assume an equal number probably refer to us as "those crazy people who dance down the street."

As I said, we always walked for half a mile per day even before the ED monster barged into our bedroom and tried to take over. We increased it to a mile to help us lose a little weight, and recently stretched that to a mile and a half. It takes us the better part of an hour now, but it's worth it. We feel better and it really does help with weight loss. And I get my husband all to myself for that time every day. We take along a cell phone for emergencies (like the house fire) and so our families can get hold of us if they need to. But typically we ignore most of the calls and just focus on each other.

Jacob jokes that walking helps with his diet mainly because he can't eat while he's so far away from the refrigerator. And while that may have (just a smidgen) of merit, the exercise we're getting, combined with other things we're doing, is working wonders.

If you're unable to have another exercise program, please consider walking. It's ideal for most people because you can walk at your own pace, and you can choose how far you want to walk. I have a friend with bad knees (like Jacob and his right knee) who started out walking to the end of her block and back, about a hundred yards or so total. She gradually increased it, and now walks a mile a day.

A couple of tips if you start a walking regimen:

- Take a bottle of water so you don't dehydrate
- Always have a cell phone
- Ease into it. If you get too ambitious and walk until you're exhausted the first time, you'll get disheartened and quit. Start out with a distance and

pace you can handle day after day and then gradually increase one or both.

- Don't look upon your daily walk as time wasted that you could be doing housework or other stuff. Instead look upon it as your "me" time... a time set aside each day to unstress, unwind, relax and be at one with nature.

-Take a can of mace with you if you have a problem with stray dogs in your neighborhood

- If that seems like a lot to carry, consider a "fanny" pack. We have one, and it carries everything quite nicely.

Okay, I know I'm starting to ramble on, so let's get to those other things we're doing quickly and then we'll move on.

Remember I told you that one of your best resources regarding the ED was the experiences of your friends? Men won't talk about ED among themselves, so that leaves us wives to do it: to commiserate, to share ideas, and to basically be an informal support group.

The same holds true of diet ideas. Your friends are your best resource. Even better than diet pills or the internet.

Don't believe me? Just ask them. I don't know of many women my age who haven't dieted at some point in their lives. Tell all your friends you want to lose a few pounds, and ask what worked for them.

And perhaps even more important, ask what didn't work.

All the things we're doing came from our friends.

- *We took all the fattening snacks out of our house. Completely. We just threw them in the garbage and vowed to buy no more.*

- *Instead of fattening snacks we now have healthy snacks, pre-cut and ready to eat. Each morning I'll cut up some broccoli or mushrooms or berries or melon and place them into a bowl in the refrigerator. These are things we both love, and they're there all day long so whenever we need a snack it's just a matter of opening the fridge and grabbing some. Boiled eggs are also good.*

- *On the counter we have a second bowl of snacks which don't have to be refrigerated. Grapes, cherries, plums or other fruits. Also pickles, cherry peppers and sugar-free chewing gum.*

- *This one is important... we do all our grocery shopping together now. That way if one of us is tempted to buy a box of Twinkies, the other is there to nix the idea. And since we almost never have cravings at the same time, this one works very well.*

- *Jacob has a sweet tooth, although he denies it. I freely admit that I have one. But here's the funny thing about having a sweet tooth: It really doesn't take a whole bowl of ice cream or a whole bag of candy to satisfy it. We've taken a daily dose of honey for years, ever since we found out that a teaspoon of locally produced honey can help with our allergies. The reasoning is that local bees eat the same pollens which cause your particular allergies. The pollens get into the honey they produce, and then into our bodies. The pollens' presence in our bodies help us build up a natural immunity to them. Then in allergy season, when the same pollens are in the air, they don't bother us as much. It seems to work, at least for us.*

Anyway, back to the sweet tooth thing: we used to take our teaspoon of honey each morning with our vitamins. Now, we just leave it on the counter. At some point during the day, whenever we crave something sweet, we take our honey. Believe it or not, just that simple teaspoon of honey is enough to satisfy our sweet tooth for awhile.

- *We haven't nixed unhealthy snacks completely. But we limit them as much as we can, and we have to earn them. For example, if one of us has an overpowering need for chocolate, we'll go to the 7-Eleven to get a candy bar. But... we have to earn it by **walking** to the 7-Eleven, we always buy the smallest bar they have, and we split it between the two of us.*

- *We tend to eat out a lot. Three times a week on average. It's not that we're not capable in the kitchen. We're both good cooks. It's just that we're at the stage in our lives when we want somebody else to do the cooking sometimes. When we eat out, we'll agree on an entrée and then we'll split it. The waitress will bring you an empty plate if you just ask. That way we get to splurge by eating what we want. We just get less of it.*

- *And we never, ever, take home leftovers. If we can't finish it all at the restaurant, we leave it there.*

- *We switched to light or low calorie foods whenever we could. Most of them taste just as good as the fattening version.*

- *Jacob likes a beer or two most nights of the week. He'd had light beers before at social gatherings and such when it was the only thing available. He made a comment that they tasted more or less the same as his brand of choice. So I said, "why not switch then?" He did and was satisfied. That led us to switch from Coke to Diet Coke, Dr. Pepper to Diet Dr. Pepper, sweetener in our coffee and iced tea instead of sugar. The days of that yucky aftertaste in diet drinks is pretty much gone. These days most diet drinks taste just as good as their sugary counterparts.*

- *We each drink a full bottle of water between dinnertime and bedtime. It helps chase away those late-night cravings which are the enemy to every diet. It also helps us stay hydrated, which is important to help our digestive systems properly process our food and get the waste quickly out of our bodies.*

- *We drink a full glass of liquid (sometimes water, sometimes iced tea, occasionally a diet soda) before each meal. We sit at the table and socialize and talk of our day, and share idle gossip, and drink a full glass of liquid before we take the first bite. That not only gives us a chance to catch up one on one, it means our stomach is already half full even before we start to eat. And it's nice, being able to just take a few minutes from our busy days and give each other our full and undivided attention.*

- *We do the same thing at restaurants, by the way, which is actually easier to do because we never ever get appetizers. By the time our entrée is cooked and served, we're typically on our second glass of drink anyway.*

I should note that these diet suggestions are much like our other suggestions to combat your erectile dysfunction. I realize that our bodies are all different, and things that worked to help Jacob and I lose a few pounds may or may not work for you. Please, consider these, and any others I haven't mentioned. Try a lot of different things, and discard those which won't work for you.

If you take away anything from this section, take these two things:

Getting and staying at or near your optimal weight will usually help with the ED problem.

Getting and staying at or near your optimal weight has benefits far beyond helping with your ED. You'll feel better, you'll have more energy, and you just might live longer.

Good luck.

Chapter 15:   *If you smoke, stop*

It's a nasty and costly habit anyway.

Smoking is like overeating in some regards.

Don't interrupt. Yes it is.

We *know* that one requires a fork and the other a lighter.

We *know* that you can smoke a steak but you can't eat a cigarette.

Well, you could, but we doubt you'd like it much.

The two are totally different things, yet have some very important things in common.

Did you know that moderate smokers (defined as ten to nineteen cigarettes a day) are four times more likely to experience serious erection problems (defined as never or seldom obtaining an erection) than men who never smoked?

And it gets even scarier.

Heavy smokers (a pack a day or higher) are nine times more likely to develop the same issues.

This study came from the Chinese, who know a thing or two about having babies. And, presumably, about having erections.

You can insert your own joke here if you want, but we did indeed mean erections, not elections.

The Chinese are famous for their efforts to limit their population growth, after crunching the numbers a generation ago. They decided that if they didn't get a handle on their growth rate, within two generations they'd have way more people than they could feed.

And since they were an extremely isolated society, they didn't like the thought of depending on other countries to feed their people.

Never mind that they're a huge country. The fact is, much of their land is unsuitable for growing crops. Much of it is permafrost. Frozen pretty much all the time. Much of it is mountain ranges. And much of it is flat and warm, but the soil is too poor or rocky to grow anything of value.

So the Chinese had to resort to other methods to solve their population-versus-food problem.

They were widely criticized in the 1980s for their one-child per household mandate. Leaders around the world called it a human rights violation. They said it was cruel to make every child in China an only child.

They said that siblings were kind of important, and not just to wear your clothes before they were handed down for you to wear.

They said that siblings help each other learn, and grow and mature. And they provide needed love and support that single children lack and will affect them later on.

Of course, all the grown-up single children around the world said that was all hogwash. That they turned out just fine.

But that didn't sway them.

Some countries (and world leaders) just aren't happy unless they're sticking their noses in somebody else's business.

Oh. You knew that. Well, okay, then.

Perhaps not coincidentally, around the same time China implemented their one-child-per-family rule, they also implemented extremely liberal abortion policies. Basically any woman who wanted to get an abortion could get one, paid for by the Chinese government, merely by asking for it.

The same woman could get another abortion six months later, and another six months after that. She could get one every six months until she reached the end of her child-bearing years if she wanted to.

The Chinese government gladly saw to her needs, and presumably said, "Thanks for coming in and doing your part to control our population. See you again in six months."

Yet the oddest thing happened.

Or rather didn't happen.

The world stayed more or less silent about the abortion policy, and continued to rail about China's one-child policy.

Oh, the Chinese did other things to help reign in its runaway growth.

They offered free sterilization surgery for those who were interested.

And they passed out condoms like they were candy. There's a now-famous photograph of two young Chinese boys blowing up condoms like balloons on a street corner. It seems they were that prevalent. One merely had to go into a market and grab a handful from a basket.

Anyway, the point of all this is that the Chinese were undergoing a huge and unwanted boom in its population, at the very same time the Chinese government was studying smoking and the effects smoking might have on erectile dysfunction (known more commonly back then as impotence).

What they found was that smoking did indeed keep a man from "getting it up."

And here's the funny thing… well, it's only funny if you're not a Chinese man… the reason the Chinese government was studying the relation of the two (smoking and impotence) to begin with was so that they could warn people to stop smoking.

But as soon as they found out for sure there was a correlation, they dropped the study like a proverbial hot potato.

It seemed they decided they no longer cared how many Chinese men would later die from lung cancer or smoke-related heart disease.

As long as the cigarettes kept the men from getting erections, they helped China's population control policy. And therefore it was okay with the Chinese government for their citizens to keep smoking away.

Nice. Real nice.

From Jacob:

I smoked my first cigarette at the tender age of seven, behind my family's back yard shed in Springfield, Missouri. My cousin Mike took two cigarettes from a pack of Camels his dad had left on the back of the toilet.

Young boys are curious by nature, and especially so when something seems dangerous or is forbidden by their parents.

Smoking was both, so we sat behind that shed one summer day and used wooden kitchen matches to light those first two smokes.

I remember several things about that experience. First, I remember coughing when the first draw of smoke seared my lungs.

Then I remember laughing it off, saying I must be coming down with something, and trying my best to look cool. I even let the thing hang from my lips, like James Dean, until it fell into my lap and burned my leg (that was back in the days when I wore shorts, before I decided my legs looked funny).

I remember my cousin Mike didn't cough as much as I did. But he turned an awful shade of green.

I didn't like it much. For one thing, because it was unfiltered and I got a mouthful of loose tobacco. I was still spitting the stuff out the next day.

Lastly, I remember wondering what in the world was the appeal? Why did adults waste their time doing something that made them cough, burned their lungs and gave them no pleasure?

I next picked up a cigarette when I was in high school, long after we'd burned the shed to the ground. (No, we weren't smoking. We were burning ants to a crisp with a magnifying glass and accidentally set the grass on fire)

In high school, skipping class and smoking weed behind the school was for stoners and losers. But smoking cigarettes in the boys' room was the ultimate in cool.

The teachers seldom went in there. We always thought they were afraid to, because some of the boys were pretty tough. We called them hoods back then. I don't know what they're called now. Gangstas, maybe.

Anyway, the second time I picked up cigarettes I picked them up to be cool. And by the time I realized I didn't need them to be cool (I was already way cool without them) I was hooked.

Over the years I tried many times to quit, for many different reasons.

In college, when I was working two jobs and eating ramen noodles and canned soup to survive, I tried to quit because I just couldn't afford them.

Actually, my plan wasn't to give them up so much as it was to quit buying them myself and to mooch cigarettes from my friends. After awhile they figured out what I was doing and quit sharing them.

During my college days I was able to slow down, but never stopped smoking completely. I even remember a couple of times skipping meals because I couldn't afford soup as well as cigarettes.

There were several times when I tried to stop to pacify the women in my life. It never took. Either the women eventually went away and I was heartbroken and went back to the cigarettes to make me feel better.

Or I decided I liked the cigarettes better than the women and sent them away, keeping the cigarettes instead.

When I met Michelle she let it be known she didn't much like me smoking, but said I was a grown man and had a right to smoke if I wanted to. At the same time, though, she told me when and if I ever wanted to quit, she'd help me as much as she could.

Over the years I tried a lot of the traditional methods to stop smoking but was not successful. Usually I could stop for a time, but went back to using them as a crutch whenever things were particularly stressful.

When I was diagnosed with erectile dysfunction, my doctor Paul said that giving up smoking was one of the best things I could do to help.

He explained his logic this way: Nobody knows why smoking affects a man's ability to get and obtain an erection. It just does. Very profound of him.

But, he says, there are also a slew of other reasons to give up smoking. Primarily, you live longer. So presumably, he says, by giving it up, you have the opportunity to live more years AND to have more sex to make those years more enjoyable.

Besides, he said, if you give up smoking and it doesn't help your ED, you've still benefitted. You still reap the other medical benefits of stopping.

I once smoked a carton of cigarettes a week and spent an average of fifty dollars a week on them. Actually, the truth was I didn't smoke all of them. But I lit that many. I had a tendency to light one, take two or three drags from it, then leave it in an ashtray to burn itself out while I went back to work or ran off to do something else.

I'd known for many years that I needed to give up the habit. As I said, I tried and failed many times before. Looking back now, though, I don't think I ever really put that much effort into quitting. Because to quit, you have to really really want it. And until you get to that point, you're playing a loser's game.

Around the same time we started studying smoking as it related to ED, I also started reading up on the dangers of second hand smoke.

Dad died when he was sixty of lung cancer. That surprised no one, because he was a long-term smoker as well. Did you know the United States Army used to actually give free cigarettes to its soldiers during World War II? Many smokers who lived in that era traced their addictions to that.

Mom died when she was 64 of emphysema and heart disease, even though she never smoked a day in her life.

If the ED connection isn't enough to sway you to quit, consider the effects of second hand smoke on your loved ones too.

When I finally told Paul I wanted to quit once and for all and needed help to do it, he referred me to another friend who specialized in addictions.

I remember walking into his office and feeling like a heroin fiend. I envisioned having to sit in a big circle of people in a large room and having to stand up and say "My name is Jacob and I'm addicted to cigarettes."

But it was nothing like that. Dave put me on a patch and sent me to a vape shop to buy a vaping rig. He also recommended I try what he called "intense dirty shoe therapy." That sounded bizarre and was not an official medical term. It's his own term, but he gave me permission to use it.

He explained that you can buy little inserts that go into the end of your cigarettes that make them taste bad. I didn't even know they existed, but he gave me a website and told me to order them.

Michelle put herself in charge of that aspect of my treatment. She ordered the inserts, which look like little slivers of wood and are about half an inch long.

Bless her little heart, she then spent hours, opening up my carton of cigarettes and then opening each pack, one by one. She shoved one of the inserts into each of the cigarettes until it disappeared, so I wouldn't be tempted to pull them back out.

And they worked like a charm. I could still light the cigarettes and take a big drag off of them, but they tasted pretty bad. Dave described the taste as smoking an old shoe. I don't know if I'd describe it the same way, but it definitely wasn't pleasant.

Michelle went with me to the vape shop and patiently waited while I tried several of the dozens of flavors they offered.

Vaping, I must say, was much more pleasant than inhaling the dirty shoe. I admit I felt kind of ridiculous puffing away on a contraption I thought made me look like a geek or a college student or both.

But there's something odd about vaping. When you start to vape you think you're the only one in the world who does it. Because you don't look for it. But once you're a vaper (as opposed to a vapor or a viper, two totally different things) you tend to notice other people doing it. You'll see them in a crowd when you never would have noticed them before. Or you'll catch a scent in the air and know that somebody is vaping the same banana nut bread flavored vape that you yourself enjoy.

Also, vaping gives you admittance into a sort of brotherhood that only vapers are welcome in.

If you're walking down the street with a vape pipe in your hand and pass another vaper, you'll nod to each other. You are brothers, of sorts. You're on the same team. He or she might even stop and ask you what you're vaping.

Michelle says if vaping continues to catch on, it'll be like the singles bars of the 1980s and 1990s. There will be vaping bars all over the country where vapers will go to find their perfect match.

I don't know about that. I think she was kidding, but with my nutty wife you never can tell.

I do know one thing, though. Vaping wasn't as bad as I thought it was. And it's not addictive, as I thought it might be. I was worried that I might trade one addiction for another, but that wasn't the case. As I sit here and type these words I can see my vape pipe across the room, lying on a table all lonely and miserable and no doubt missing my sweet lips. It's been there, untouched, for about four days now.

Those are the three things that helped me quit.

The patch (which has to be prescribed), the stinky shoe inserts, and the vape.

Actually, I need to add a couple more: the choice between dying sooner or getting a boner and having sex more often. A no-brainer, really.

And the support and help of a great woman.

Michelle is standing behind me, hands on her hips, demanding, "And just who the hell is this great woman you're talking about?"

It is, of course, my incredibly lovely wife Michelle. She's my one and only and always will be.

This was by far the most difficult thing I've done in years, either before or after we started our "Ed Project." I cheated many times, sneaking a cigarette when I thought I could get away with it.

Finally, I realized I was only cheating myself. Of a longer life, a fuller sex life.

If you're a smoker and you decide to quit, either to help your ED or for any other reason, don't give up. It's an addiction not much different from cocaine or heroin. It has withdrawal symptoms just like the harshest drug, and you'll find yourself actually hungering for cigarettes. Especially in times of stress.

One thing I'd like to leave you with: if you break down and smoke a cigarette occasionally, don't beat yourself up. And even more importantly, don't use that as an excuse to give up. Many people do, figuring, "Well, I've failed. Might as well start smoking again."

No. Don't. Just recognize that you've taken a single step back on a long journey, and then move forward again. You can do this. I know you can.

From Michelle:

When Jacob told me he was going to quit smoking to aid us in what we'd begun calling "Project Ed" I was ecstatic.

Then it occurred to me that I'd heard it all before.

I've never smoked. Not even once. I'm not saying that to sound smug or to brag. I just never had the desire to try.

My best girlfriend in high school once offered me one and I asked her, "Why? What's the point?" She thought for a moment, couldn't find an answer to my question, and snuffed out her cigarette. I wish I could tell you she stopped then and there, but she didn't. She was already hooked.

She died four years ago of heart disease. She was only fifty four years of age.

Jacob knew early on I didn't approve of his smoking. I told him on our first or second date that kissing him was like emptying an ash tray full of cigarette ashes into my mouth and chewing on them.

One of the tenets our relationship is built on is to respect one another and their choices, and to not try to change the other. He knew I didn't approve, but I never pushed it. So he continued to do it.

He smoked his last cigarette about four months ago. He recently made a comment I found interesting. He was sitting in the incredibly ugly recliner he's had for years and said, "Honey, we need to get rid of this chair."

I asked why and he said, "Because it smells like an ashtray. It's sickening."

I told him, "Honey, that's how the whole house used to smell" (still does, but it's fading).

I said, "You just never noticed it before. But the smell of burned cigarettes used to permeate everything. Your clothes, our walls, even me. You never noticed it before because it permeated you."

We'll never know to what degree his not smoking anymore has helped with his ED. That's the most maddening thing about this whole process. When you try a combination of things to fix a problem, you don't necessarily know which one or ones fixed the problem and which ones fell flat. That's why we're giving you so many options in your "tool box." And why we encourage you to try them all, and to find your own tools, and to keep trying until you find the right combination that works for you.

I will say this though... he needed to stop for a variety of reasons.

And I'm glad he did. Every time he slips his hard penis inside me I'm even more glad.

Oh, and he tastes much better when he kisses me now. I'll admit I'd forgotten what joy it was to kiss a man who didn't smoke. I'm sure glad I got that (and other things) back into my life.

Erectile Dysfunction Tool Box Thus Far: 17 Items

1. Frequent penis stimulation
2. Pin stimulation to penis head
3. Eat well. Diet is everything
4. Enlist your doctor's help
5. A good selection of written erotica
6. Play. Experiment. Find new things to love
7. Water is our friend. Drink lots of it.
8. Limit caffeine
9. Ice can be nice
10. Try warming oils as a stimulant
11. Porn as a visual mood setter
12. ED Medications as a backup, not as a go-to
13. Learn to save some for a rainy day
14. Change the mechanics of how you make love
15. Whack your wiener for her. She'll enjoy it and it'll help with the ED
16. Lose those extra pounds. It'll help too
17. If you smoke, stop no matter how hard it is

Chapter 16: *Get your prostate checked*

It's something you need to keep your eye on anyway.

Okay, let's face it… getting older really sucks.

It's hard enough as we pass fifty and near our "golden years," as we discover the golden years aren't so golden after all.

We develop pain in joints we weren't smart enough to take care of when we were younger, and in muscles we didn't even know existed.

Our eyesight and hearing start to wane and we have to start wearing reading glasses just to read the daily paper.

And our mailbox starts filling with mailers we never asked for, never wanted, and don't even know how they knew we'd turned old.

Junk mail from companies specializing in arthritis treatment, dentures, walkers and wheelchairs, and all kinds of other stuff to remind us we're not the spring chickens we once were.

One of the biggest things men have to deal with as we grow older is an enlarged prostate.

It's a major pain.

For the first time in our lives, we have to make a decision before we go to bed. Do we really want to quench our thirst with that last glass of water, knowing we'll be up at least twice during the night to urinate?

Or do we forego the water and go to bed with a dry mouth and thirst pangs, just to try to get a good night's sleep?

If you're over fifty and still able to sleep through the night, count yourself lucky. Then look up to the sky and thank your long-dead Grandfather Stanley, for blessing you with good genes.

Lastly, cross your fingers and hope your luck holds.

Because you're very unusual.

Most men over fifty aren't so lucky. Most men over fifty have to get up once, twice, three times during the night to urinate.

Most men over fifty haven't had a good night's sleep in years.

They stumble out of bed, head to the bathroom, whip that sucker out, and then curse under their breath because they don't get the healthy stream of urine they need to empty their swollen and aching bladder.

Instead they get a trickle or a drip.

It's caused by an enlarged prostate. You probably already know that.

But here are some things you may not know.

A lot of men (you may be one of them) just presume that an enlarged prostate and problems with urination (either too frequent or not frequent enough) is an unavoidable part of getting older. Those men may think that since their father had the same problem, and their grandfather before him, that he must suffer as well.

Pay his dues like the other males in his family, so to speak.

But that's not the case. An enlarged prostate can be treated.

That's why you should consult your physician.

Let's say you're one of those stubborn men who refuse to go to the doctor unless you actually see blood or lose consciousness.

Hopefully you're not. But there are an awful lot of men out there who are that way.

Or… let's say you're one of those men who don't have health insurance and have to budget for your doctor's visits. You save up your complaints until you have several of them and then go see your doctor about all of them at once.

Hopefully you're not one of these men either, but there are an awful lot of them out there too.

All is not lost for you two groups of men.

You don't have to see a doctor to treat your enlarged prostate. Of course, that's always the best option. But if you choose not to for whatever reason, there are plenty of non-prescription and natural remedies on the market.

Here's a partial list, although there are many more:

- Saw Palmetto
- Beta Sitosteral
- Pygeum
- Rye Grass Pollen
- Stinging Nettle
- Foods high in zinc and vitamin C

We are NOT recommending for or against any of these products. What works for one may not work for another. You should also know that the American Urological Association does not recommend herbal therapy for an enlarged prostate. They'd prefer you see your physician. So would we. But we're going to put this information out there anyway for you hard-heads. If you want to try any of these, you can find them at your local health or natural food store.

As with all things you put into your body, though, you must do your homework and practice due diligence.

Okay, some of you who aren't the fastest gunslinger in the old west might be asking why we're talking about treating an enlarged prostate, when the real reason you're here is because you have a problem with ED.

It's because the two are related.

A lot of men who sought treatment for their enlarged prostate, or who were able to lessen its effects by altering their diets or adding natural supplements, noticed a reduction in their problems getting and keeping an erection.

That's why we're talking about this.

From Jacob:

My doctor and good friend Paul was the one who told me there was a connection between my enlarged prostate and my erectile dysfunction. I hadn't a clue.

Paul isn't like a normal doctor.

One of the things I like about him, (besides that he's a lousy bowler and I consistently beat him by twenty pins or better) is that he's always hesitant to prescribe medication when other things might work.

He suggested I try Saw Palmetto to ease my prostate issues, and it seemed to help me. When I told him so he said we'd consider the problem solved unless it came back.

Then a little later, when I told him I was having problems getting erections, the very first thing he asked me was "Is your prostate bothering you again?"

It seems that men with prostate problems often develop ED, although it doesn't work the other way around.

Simply put, if you're having trouble urinating, or are urinating frequently, AND you're having ED issues, you can frequently ease the ED problem by treating your prostate.

I should note here that frequent urination can also be an indicator of diabetes, which can also cause ED or make it worse.

Your best bet is to see your physician if you're having problems with urination (either going too little or going too often). If your doctor is on the ball, he'll test you for diabetes, and will ask if you've had problems with intimacy.

As I said, it's all kind of tied in together.

Paul is a doctor who'd prefer his patients forego prescription drugs when natural treatments work better. He told me on the golf course last weekend about a long-time patient (he didn't mention names, that would be unethical) who came to him in a panic. The patient insisted on getting referred for lap-band surgery to lose forty nagging pounds.

Paul refused his request and sent him to a dietician instead.

"You don't need surgery," he told the man. "You just need to eat better and smarter."

Many physicians would have leapt at the chance to refer this patient to a friend who did lap-band surgeries. But Paul's not that way. He's on the side of his patients, not his surgical buddies or pharmacological reps.

He printed me out a list of natural and herbal remedies for enlarged prostate.

"Try these first. They're available at your natural foods store, and some won't work for you at all. Others might work well. If none of them relieve your prostate problems, then we'll consider prescribing you something."

It turned out that for me, the Saw Palmetto was all I needed. Your results may vary.

The point is this… if you're having urination issues anyway, you need to look into it, whether you're having erection issues or not. If you're having erection issues also, then you have twice as many reasons to get your prostate checked.

Quit making excuses and just do it.

Chapter 17:   *While we're talking natural remedies...*

Try these to help with your ED

There's an old saying that goes something like "You are what you eat." Come on, you know you've heard it. Jacob even had a t-shirt emblazoned with the saying back in the 1970s, before he finally developed a sense of fashion.

He wore it with his bell bottoms and poncho and Greek sandals.

He also had a sky blue leisure suit, but that was for special occasions.

Here's a surprising thing about that old saying. It's largely true.

You really are what you eat.

The human body, you see, is a product of what you put into it. Some of it is absorbed through sunlight. But not much. Most of it is derived by things that go into our mouth and are swallowed.

We, therefore, have a greater say-so than anybody on the state of our body at any given time. We are the masters and mistresses of our own universe.

Well, maybe not. But we're certainly the masters and mistresses of our own design.

Consider this: we have a choice whether to be healthy.

Someone who is extremely health-conscious and wants to try to live forever will eat only healthy foods. Foods that are rich in proteins and vitamins. Their diet will be mostly vegetarian, but they'll make room for a limited amount of lean meats and eggs. They'll never, ever, put sugar into their bodies, or caffeine, or fat, or things like carbohydrates which will turn into sugar and then fat.

And they'll likely have a very miserable, albeit very healthy, life.

On the other hand, someone who doesn't care very much whether they drop dead at age fifty will gorge on junk food. They'll be a two-fisted eater, with a big greasy cheeseburger in one hand and a slice of pizza in the other.

They'll eat a one pound bag of M&Ms each and every day of their lives and will wash it down with sugared soda and beer. No water, ever. Just sugared soda and beer. They'll stay up all night being a keyboard warrior on their computer or watch old movies on television, swigging a bottle of whiskey and complaining they can't sleep because of indigestion.

They'll likely live a leisurely and relatively happy existence.

But they won't live very long.

The vast majority of us aren't like the ultra-fit healthy guy or the out-of shape eating machine.

We're somewhere in the middle.

We try to live a relatively healthy lifestyle. We make an effort to get off the couch and get some exercise occasionally. We even try to lose those few extra pounds, although we're just as likely to do it to keep our doctors off our backs than to gain any health benefits from it.

And we, as free-thinking adults, are the ones who decide which foods and beverages we place into our bodies.

Recognizing that, we're not going to bore you with a long list of the foods you should eat more of. To find those out, you merely have to pick up one of the popular magazines. You've seen them at the supermarket checkout. Their covers are constantly touting headlines like *10 Foods You Should Be Eating*, or *Eat Healthier. Here's How*.

The point is, we literally *are* what we eat. It's our choice, and no one else's.

But this isn't a diet book, nor is it a healthy lifestyle book.

This is a book to help you combat your erectile dysfunction.

And while those three things (healthy lifestyle, diet and battling ED) go hand in hand to some degree, we're focusing on your bedroom activities.

So we're not giving you a list of foods to make you lose weight or live ten extra years.

We're giving you a list of foods which may help your ED.

And we're betting you didn't know there was such a list, did you?

Well there is. There's nothing scientific about it, really. Although there have been many studies conducted to determine the relation between the types of foods we eat and male impotence, there's never been a list published (to our knowledge) by the scientific or medical communities to recommend certain foods to combat ED.

Until now.

As far as we know, we're the first.

Ta-dah!

To be honest, we didn't assemble this list for you, our readers. We assembled it for Jacob, to help bring back his erections. But it seemed to work for him. To what degree, we'll never know, since we were trying so many other things at the same time.

We'll never know to what degree eating cashews helped give him that erection, and how much was the penis pump we were also using that night. The point is we did a lot of research over the past months. And we've compiled a list of foods and herbal things which studies have shown had a positive impact on a man's ability to get and keep an erection.

Here is that list.

- oysters
- beef
- crab
- lobster
- cashews
- chickpeas
- breakfast cereals (the ones which say "fortified")
- chicken
- Swiss cheese
- oatmeal
- cottage cheese
- almonds
- kidney beans

Here's a second list of herbal remedies. Some of these may not be available in your area, and some can only be found at health food stores or on-line.

And some of them didn't seem to have any effect on Jacob at all.

Again, it seems to go back to that "every man is different" mantra. What works on John might not work at all on Joe.

But here's the list if you want to try any of them.

- Asian ginseng
- Arginine
- DHEA
- Korean Red ginseng
- Pomegranate juice

- Yohimbe
- Goat weed (Icariin)
- Ginko Biloba

From Jacob:

Paul, my doctor, was a bit leery when I told him I wanted to try goat weed and some of the other stuff.

He told me to only use things I obtained from a legitimate source, so I'll pass that advice onto you, our readers.

In other words, if you can find these things on the shelf at a health food store or for sale from a reputable on-line source, great.

Don't buy them from a guy named Rico, from the back of his beat up van, in a dark alley somewhere.

And don't buy them from a strange-looking internet site you probably shouldn't trust either. Instead of getting goat weed you might be getting dandelion leaves.

And if you want dandelion leaves, we've got a whole bunch in our front yard I can't seem to get rid of. Help yourself to as many as you want.

The point is, our body is our temple. Treat it as such. Feel free to try these things, but in limited quantities until you find out whether you're allergic to them or whether they're of any benefit to you.

I tried to sample all of the herbals. Some of them I just couldn't find. I also tried to include at least one of the food items in every meal.

It really helped that I happen to love seafood and shellfish, which make up a good portion of the items on the food list.

I never ate a lot of chicken, and I'm ashamed to say most of the time I did eat it, it was fried.

Michelle, on the other hand, loves chicken, and since we started this endeavor has been experimenting with new recipes.

There must be a thousand different ways to make chicken. And at least a couple of hundred are not only tasty, but relatively healthy as well. She made a baked chicken dish with sliced vegetables and lime juice a week ago that still makes my mouth water. It was friendly to my diet and to my heart. Whether it made my dick hard, I don't know for sure. But we did make love for well over an hour that night.

Here's my advice on this list of foods.

If you see something on the list you like, try to eat more of it. If you see something on the list you've never tried, try it. As we always told our kids when they were young (and still tell our grandkids), if you never try new things, you'll never find new things you love.

Bear in mind that some people are allergic to shell fish, so if you've never tried them, go easy at first.

And if you just don't like something on the list, go on to something else.

From Michelle:

As we've said from the beginning, it's hard for us to point the finger at any one thing and say, "That's it! That's the thing that cured Jacob's ED!" because we're doing lots of things at the same time.

I will say that getting him hard is a lot easier now that we're eating more of these foods.

Most of the things on this list have the added benefit of being relatively healthy, and many of them are relatively low calorie was well. So it might be the combination: that these things are known to help with

ED, that they're helping Jacob (and me too) lose weight, and they're giving Jacob (and me too) more energy that is helping with our ED problem.

Erectile Dysfunction Tool Box Thus Far: 19 Items

1. Frequent penis stimulation
2. Pin stimulation to penis head
3. Eat well. Diet is everything
4. Enlist your doctor's help
5. A good selection of written erotica
6. Play. Experiment. Find new things to love
7. Water is our friend. Drink lots of it.
8. Limit caffeine
9. Ice can be nice
10. Try warming oils as a stimulant
11. Porn as a visual mood setter
12. ED Medications as a backup, not as a go-to
13. Learn to save some for a rainy day
14. Change the mechanics of how you make love
15. Whack your wiener for her. She'll enjoy it and it'll help with the ED
16. Lose those extra pounds. It'll help too
17. If you smoke, stop no matter how hard it is
18. Check your prostate
19. Look hard at the foods you're eating

Chapter 18:   *Avoid the blame game*

Stress is the biggest mood killer of all

Since Jacob was diagnosed with erectile dysfunction we've been careful not to consider it his problem.

It was "our" problem from the beginning. We accepted it as such and decided to attack it as a team.

We decided we were going to work together to kick ED's ass, and we've been able to do that.

And after all, it just makes sense. After all, why consider it just the man's problem when it adversely affects both of us?

We both love sex. We always have. The thought of living the rest of our lives without it was inconceivable to us and something we just weren't willing to accept.

You both love sex as well. If you didn't, you wouldn't be reading these words right now.

So we beg of you... since you love sex and want to get it back, don't fall into a vicious trap we call "the blame game."

From Michelle:

Since we started this project we've spoken to a lot of people about ED, its origins, and its affects, not only on his ability to get it up, but the psychological impact on both parties.

Maybe it was because we decided to fight it together from the beginning, but we were amazed at how many couples let themselves be divided over this issue.

One of my good friends (I'll call her Mary, although that's not her real name) confided that her husband of many years had a major problem with ED.

I never had a clue. They were a happy couple in every other way, or at least appeared to be.

When I told her that Jacob and I were working on this project an odd look came over her face. I knew in my heart she and "Bill" were suffering the same problem Jacob and I were.

But it took her awhile to open up about it. She finally admitted to me that she was ashamed. Not for herself, but for her husband.

"I didn't want the word to get out that he has this problem."

That **he** *had the problem. He, as is he alone.*

It turned out that Mary and Bill's once vibrant sex life had trickled away to nothing, and she was blaming him for it.

Oh, she wasn't mean about it at all. She didn't yell at him or belittle him for his inability to get an erection. She chose instead to ignore it. To never talk about it. To stop fondling her husband. To give up on sex altogether. And that, of course, made the situation much worse.

Because that's the worst thing you can possibly do.

Bill already felt bad about the situation. He was already under a lot of stress, feeling inadequate and unable to pleasure his wife of many years. He already felt he was somewhat less of a man than he'd been in previous years.

Here's something you may not have realized: such feelings increase stress for both parties. And stress makes the problem so much worse.

Don't either of you blame the other.

And just as important, don't either of you blame yourselves. It's nobody's fault. Really.

Chapter 19:   *Don't Do Without, Guys, For Any Extended Period.*

That's what did us in...

From Michelle:

We believe the main reason the ED monster came around was because Jacob was totally abstinent when he was abroad. And by totally abstinent I mean he wasn't even jerking off.

I knew he jerked off occasionally during our marriage. I heard him whacking his wiener occasionally as I walked past the bathroom door. It wasn't often, as he much preferred sex with me. It was usually just a matter of convenience, such as when he was especially horny but had to leave for work in half an hour.

Or when I had a cold and wasn't feeling especially frisky and he didn't want to burden me.

I accepted that he jerked off occasionally over the years, and it didn't bother me in the least. Heck, who was I to talk? I fingered myself all the time when he wasn't around, and I've always had a pretty impressive collection of vibrators in what he calls my "toy drawer."

So it wouldn't have bothered me in the least if he was spanking his monkey daily while he was abroad. In fact, knowing what we know now, I'd have called him up every day to demand it.

Jacob: Hello
Me: Hi honey. Have you strangled your chicken today?

Jacob: Have I what?

Me: Have you strangled your chicken? That's what they call it nowadays. I saw it on one of those teen movies.

Jacob: Honey, it's three in the morning here.

Me: I know, dear. That's why I waited to call you until now. Don't you remember, three in the morning is when you usually get hard. If I had a dollar for every time over the years you pressed that thing against my leg, hoping I'd wake up and climb on top of you...

Jacob: But honey, I have a book signing at nine a.m. I have to get some sleep so I can be nice to my readers and get them to buy more of my books. If I'm grouchy they'll go buy somebody else's books instead. And I'll have to get a job at a 7-Eleven. You don't want me to have to get a job at a 7-Eleven, do you?

Me: (thinking) I don't know. Maybe. Would you give me free Slurpees?

Jacob: But baby, I don't want to work at a 7-Eleven. I want to write my novels. It's what I do best.

Me: It's not the only thing you do well. I know you're pretty darn good at stroking that salami too. And it's a very nice salami, by the way.

Jacob: I know what you're trying to do.

Me: What?

Jacob: You're thinking that by complimenting my salami you'll wake him up and make him hard, and then I'll have to masturbate to make him go back to sleep.

Me: Well, he does like it when I talk about him.

Jacob: (sighing) Yes, he does.

Me: So, is it working? Is he getting hard?

Jacob (sighing again) Yes.

Me: Good. I'll get off the phone now so you can butter your bread.

Jacob: Where do you come up with all these terms for masturbating?

Me: Some from movies. Some from the internet. Some I just make up. Now get to whacking, big boy.

Jacob: But I'm soooo tired.

Me: But honey, you know what Paul said. If you don't ejaculate on a regular basis while you're overseas, you may lose the ability to get a boner. Your balls will think you're no longer interested, and will stop producing semen. And remember, he said your cock is a muscle, and just like any other muscle it needs to be exercised. Otherwise it'll just go limp and just hang there. So get off the phone and slide that trombone, sweet cheeks.

Jacob: You're really enjoying this, aren't you?

Me: Immensely. But you know what I'll enjoy more?

Jacob: Sticking bamboo shoots under my fingernails?

Me: No, silly. I'll enjoy it more when you come home and get stiff as a board and slide that thing inside of me where it belongs. But that may not happen if you don't tickle the eel while you're over there.

Jacob: Can't I go back to sleep and wait until after my book signing?

Me: Absolutely not.

Jacob: But why?

Me: Because. You're in Paris. The most romantic city in the world. And I know what will happen.

Jacob: What, pray tell, will happen?

Me: If you don't beat the weasel, you'll go to your book signing and this hot French chick named Fifi will bring you a book to sign, And she'll tell you she's read every one of your books and she's always loved your work, and how my, what big muscles you have.

And she'll talk you into going back to her place and slipping your big Italian sausage into her and depositing your load there. And she doesn't deserve it. She doesn't pick up your dirty socks from the bedroom floor and cook you chicken spaghetti for your birthday like I do.

Jacob: Good story. You should be a writer or something.

Me: Ha, ha. My point is that you need to cum on a regular basis while you're there so your balls don't start to shut down. It's use it or lose it time, buddy. And I'd much rather you blow your load into the bathroom sink than in some hot chick named Fifi.

Jacob: (sighing a third time) If I get up and jerk off will you let me go back to sleep after?

Me: Of course, honey. Now get up and knead that dough. I love you so much.

Jacob: I love you too, honey. (sighing)

Me: Oh, and baby?

Jacob: Yes?

Me: I'll talk to you tomorrow morning. I'll call you about this time again...

Sorry, I got off track a little bit.

The point I was trying to make was that we firmly believe the main reason Jacob developed ED was because of the long period of time he went without sex (even masturbation). Had we known that ahead of time, he certainly would have taken precautions. But since we didn't, he didn't. And that led to a lot of unnecessary guilt on his part.

As Paul puts it:

"Guilt when it comes to ED is a never-ending circle of bad. B-A-D. Bad. What happens is that a guy will start to develop problems getting an erection. So

he feels guilty. And that leads to stress. And stress is one of the primary things that keep a man from getting an erection. So it's a vicious cycle. You have to find a way to stop that guilt, so you can reduce that stress. Then you'll increase the chances of defeating the ED dilemma."

If we'd known before Jacob went to Europe that a lack of sex would lead to his onset of ED, we'd have done things differently. I'd have encouraged him to masturbate every day while he was there. I would have even given him permission to spend time with Fifi or to dally with a French prostitute (maybe the same thing) if that's what it took.

From Jacob:

Now you tell me... sheesh.

From Michelle:

Oh shut up, you.

Anyway, we've always known that stress was a real mood killer in the bedroom, even for couples who have no problem getting hard. You know that too. We've all had times when one of us is in the mood for sex, but the other had a bad day at the office, or ran over a land mine on the way home, or something else which caused them stress.

But who knew that same stress could be a killer of penises?

I should note here and now that guilt works both ways. For awhile after he returned from Europe

Jacob suffered in silence. He was moody and irritable and sulked a lot. He kept to himself, and when I asked what was the matter he always said, "nothing."

Looking back, I was sure it was just the ED. It was new to us at that time and we panicked. We didn't know what caused it or how to fix it and we thought it was permanent. We thought our sex life was over forever.

And Jacob blamed himself, in silence. Now I feel awful because I didn't know what he was feeling, didn't know how to help him.

And of course, like Paul said, his feelings of guilt and of stress made the problem worse.

I should also note that I was going through the same feelings of guilt about the same time. I hid it better, because us women are always better at hiding such things.

But I remember looking in the full length mirror on our closet door one afternoon. This was after our third or fourth night of trying to make Jacob's dick hard with no success at all.

I looked in the mirror, examining my body, and shamed myself into thinking it was my fault. That I was no longer attractive. That I no longer turned him on.

I remembered the times early in our relationship when all I had to do was walk past him naked on my way to the shower, and his dick would rise within seconds. And he'd say, "Your shower can wait," and throw me onto the bed and we'd make love.

I wondered at what point I stopped being a turn-on for him and became ugly.

The twenty extra pounds I'd picked up over the years looked like a thousand and twenty.

And I swear I counted every wrinkle on my face, dozens of times. I'd have counted the gray hairs too, but I couldn't see the ones on the back of my head.

The next day I went to the mall and to Macy's. I bought a dozen different products, from cold creams to facial scrubs to relaxing lotions. I spent four hundred dollars, but I was gonna look damn good for my husband.

That same afternoon I had my hair colored for the first time in my life.

Within a week I had given up. The wrinkles were there to stay, and I didn't like my new hair color. Neither did Jacob, by the way. He told me I was as beautiful as I was the day he met me, and that I shouldn't change a single thing about the way I looked.

They were pretty words, and oh so sweet. But I didn't buy it.

I blamed myself that he couldn't get it up anymore. I convinced myself I'd become a hideous old hag. I lay in bed at night looking at the ceiling thinking I'd failed him. More than once I cried myself to sleep.

Yet I did the same thing he did. I remained silent about it. When he asked me what was wrong I said "nothing." We should have been talking it out. Reassuring each other about our continued attraction and our love for each other.

Instead we grew more and more isolated.

Other than not working his dick when he was abroad, the guilt and stress thing was the biggest mistake we made in regards to fixing OUR erectile dysfunction problem.

I hope you're not making the same mistake.

Don't play the blame game, please. It's a very bad thing.

From Jacob:

In the first weeks following my return from Europe I felt like the lowest person on earth. I felt I was no longer a man. I felt I let my wife down. I was actually worried that if I could no longer please her in the bedroom, she might look for someone else. After all, sex had always been a very important part of our lives, right up until the day I left for Europe.

It sounds ridiculous now, but I was in a very bad place then. My penis was part of my body, not hers. Therefore it was something I did to break it.

I was desperate to fix it, yet I didn't know how.

And she's right. I was very moody. I wasn't sleeping well at night. All I could think of was that I was letting her down. The only woman in the whole world I loved and I could no longer perform for her. When she asked what she could do to help I brushed her off. It was hard for me to talk about. I felt totally inadequate and totally emasculated.

I felt, in a word, like crap.

But being a typical guy, it never occurred to me that she might be feeling the same things.

I'm like most guys, I think, when I say I'm attuned to my wife's feelings.

And I am, insofar as I can tell when she's in a bad mood or when something is bothering her. I mean, that much is easy to see. She gets quiet, she snaps at me sometimes, and she isolates herself. She goes off to the den and curls up in her favorite easy chair. Then she covers herself with a quilt and reads for hours at a time.

So I know when something is wrong. Figuring out what it is, however, is a bit more difficult.

Michelle, like me, isn't very forthcoming.

That's why it took us a full week before we figured out that we were being defeated by the same kinds of feelings, and then decided to work together to stop them.

I thought the ED was all my fault. She thought it was her fault.

It wasn't until we sat down one evening in front of the fireplace and snuggled (still my all-time favorite thing to do, even after all these years) that we came clean.

Then we cried. It felt so good to get those feelings out.

Then we decided that the guilt was getting us nowhere. That we had to do as much research as we could, and try everything we needed to do, to get this problem under control

And we never looked back.

If either of you, or both of you, are feeling such guilt, stop it right now. Such feelings are only making your problems worse.

It's nobody's fault. Really.

Chapter 20:   *This just in...*

Consider a penis pump

We were getting ready to wrap this up and send it for editing, but decided to throw this in because we've had some success with it.

A few weeks ago we stumbled across something called a "penis pump" while shopping on-line for a new vibrator.

We figured, "What the heck? We can always use another tool in our toolbox." So we ordered one. It came in about two weeks ago.

From Jacob:

It's a simple device, really. It has a tube into which a man inserts his flaccid penis, and a pumping device which helps encourage blood to fill it by essentially "sucking" the blood into it.

Once the penis is filled with blood and erect, a small band (ours is rubber but some are elastic) is placed around the base of the penis to discourage the blood from escaping too fast.

I have to admit, I felt ridiculous the first time I did this. But I also admit that it worked long enough for Michelle and I to enjoy a great round of intercourse.

Maybe "session" is a better term. "Round" makes it sound like golf, and intercourse is way more fun.

Anyway, we were trying other things at the time, so the pump probably didn't do it all by itself. I don't want to lead anyone on, or make anyone think the pump is a miracle cure. But in conjunction with the other things we did that night, my penis was as hard as it was thirty years ago.

Having said that, the next time we tried it three nights later the results weren't quite so great. It got hard enough to have intercourse, but it was a bit of a struggle.

The third time we used it, the results were somewhere between the first two. It wasn't quite as hard as it was the first time, but pretty close.

The point is, the penis pump (at least in my mind) shouldn't be used as a stand-alone means of obtaining and keeping an erection. In such a capacity, it would likely fail as often as not.

However, used in conjunction with other things (like porn in the background, extended fondling or some of the other things we've talked about), I think it's a good tool.

From Michelle:

Jacob didn't want to use the pump in front of me at first. He said he felt silly.

I asked him why and he said because when he was a teenager he stuck his dick in a vacuum cleaner to get himself off.

I asked him why in the world he did that, and he said that teenage boys are so fascinated with their dicks they experiment with all kinds of things. Basically, he said, they put it anywhere and everywhere to see what feels good and what doesn't.

I asked him whether the vacuum cleaner felt good and he said it did. But that for a long time after that he felt kind of dirty, like he was a "freak" for having done it.

He said those feelings eventually went away and he pretty much forgot about it. But sticking his cock into the penis pump brought back the memory and the feelings.

I told him there was no reason to feel foolish. That we all did silly things when we were young to pleasure ourselves. And I reminded him about the time when we were in college and he walked into my dorm room and told me he had a surprise for me.

But I had to strip naked and lay back and close my eyes.

I was a bit apprehensive when he went into the hallway and brought a large cooler into the room, but I played his silly game.

Not knowing quite what to expect, I was a bit surprised to feel something very cold plop down between my breasts (which in those days were rather perky and still stood up when I was lying down).

The cold plop was followed by a series of other sensations. Finally he told me to open my eyes, and I laughed when I saw he'd built a banana split on my tits.

He only brought one spoon and we shared the banana split, with him spoon feeding me. Between bites be ran the back of the cold spoon around and around on my nipples, and I was quite turned on by the time we finished and he licked the remaining ice cream off of me.

The point I was trying to make to him was that the things we sometimes do in the name of sex is sometimes silly.

But that doesn't mean it's not fun, or worth the silliness.

Then I offered to take over the pump for him.

I've always been one to experiment, and have showed Jacob many pleasurable things over the years (like using one of my vibrators on his dick head to make him cum). So I was just chomping at the bits to use the pump on him.

As he said, we had mixed results. Sometimes it worked better than others. Use it not as a stand-alone cure-all, but rather use it at the same time you're doing other things.

From Jacob:

From the beginning of this project, one of the things we've tried not to do is to endorse any one product. Nor to advocate against something.

We figured we're not doing this on behalf of any particular company or industry. We're doing this for you, our readers, so that you can benefit from our experience.

In line with that thinking, we're not going to identify the specific penis pump we bought, nor the name of its manufacturer.

From what we saw, they all work pretty much the same way. If you choose to add one of these to your toolbox, we suggest you pick out one you like. Make sure you're comfortable with it, and that it'll accommodate your penis size.

From Michelle:

As I said, this is something I enjoy doing to him immensely. No, I don't know why. I suppose it's for the same reason I love to play with his dick. Because it gives him pleasure and at the same time helps with the ED thing.

In our house, I am the designated "Queen of the penis pump." I crowned myself. He is no longer allowed to use it on himself. That's my job. He says he much prefers when I do it and it's a bigger turn-on than when he applies it himself.

And, as we all well know, the bigger the turn-on the more (and bigger) the erections.

My suggestion, ladies, is that you all take control of the penis pump for the very same reason.

IN CONCLUSION...

There are several very important things we want to leave you with.

1) What works for one man might not work for another. Remember our snowflake analogy. No two men are alike. That's why it's imperative you don't just try one thing and then give up when it doesn't work. You must try many things until you find out which ones work for you.

2) What works for you tonight might not necessarily work for you next week or next month. If one of your tried and true methods suddenly stops working for you, don't freak out or give up. Simply try other methods in your toolbox until you find something else that is working with you.

3) Using just one method usually isn't successful. Use a variety of things, in conjunction with one another, to achieve your best erection. Because you never know which one may or may not be working on a particular night. You wouldn't eat just one M&M and expect to be satisfied. So why would you settle for just one ED tool?

4) Wives, talk to your friends. Tell them in confidence that your husband is having problems getting hard. You will be truly amazed at how many of their husbands are having difficulties as well. Then, once you've established that common ground, share ideas.

Tell them what works for you, and ask them what worked for them. Your husbands will not do this. You must, therefore, do it yourself. Husbands are all big and bad when it comes to talking sports. But when it comes to discussing their ED problems with their male friends, they're sissies. This is one of your BEST sources to get additional tools for your toolbox. Don't pass it up.

Along those lines, we're going to give you one last copy of our completed toolbox. The back of it will be blank, so you can tear it out of the book.

We'd like for you to tear it out and place it in your bedroom where it'll be handy.

After awhile, you'll find which tools work for you, or which ones you prefer using. Until you get to that point, though, you might need an occasional memory jogger. Every single item we list in our toolbox worked for us. Some to a great degree and some to lesser degrees. But every one of them worked, and we firmly believe they'll work for you too.

Granted, there is some stigma attached to some of them.

But consider this: Stigma is your second worst enemy, after the ED itself.

If you let stigma prevent you from trying something you're a bit shy or squeamish about, you might miss out on the very thing that works best for you.

In other words, kick stigma to the curb. Go into this adventure with a completely open mind. Try anything and everything at least once. If you determine it didn't work, or just wasn't a good fit for you, then discard it and try something else. But everything you flat refuse to try might be a missed opportunity.

Or a missed solution.

Sharing of ideas is the main way we will help solve the ED problem for millions of couples. Medication is a wonderful thing. But it isn't the magical solution. Many people cannot take ED medication for a variety of health or other reasons. Or because they just don't work for them.

That's the bad news.

The good news is that there are a lot of other things that can work.

We want to hear your own stories. We want to hear what worked for you, and what didn't. As you talk to your friends and share ideas, you'll find your own tools to put in your toolbox that perhaps we haven't tried yet.

We want you to share those with us too.

Most of you are on Facebook now. Please send us a friend request and tell us how you're coming. Our Facebook page is JacobandMichelle Clark. If you're not on Facebook, that's okay. You can just email us at JacobandMichelleClark@yahoo.com

Also, we'd like to do a sequel to this book, so we can get even more ideas out there fo r the millions of couples who need help.

Those of you who want to share your stories can be included in the book. We'll use first names only, and can even use pseudonyms if you prefer. If you find something which works for you that we didn't cover, help us get the word out. Everybody likes a good success story, and sharing them is especially rewarding when you know you're helping others.

The sequel will be called *Erectile Dysfunction: What Worked For Our Friends*. We're looking forward to writing it.

Jacob and Michelle's Erectile Dysfunction Tool Box: 21 Items

1. Frequent penis stimulation
2. Pin stimulation to penis head
3. Eat well. Diet is everything
4. Enlist your doctor's help
5. A good selection of written erotica
6. Play. Experiment. Find new things to love
7. Water is our friend. Drink lots of it.
8. Limit caffeine
9. Ice can be nice
10. Try warming oils as a stimulant
11. Porn as a visual mood setter
12. ED Medications as a backup, not as a go-to
13. Learn to save some for a rainy day
14. Change the mechanics of how you make love
15. Whack your wiener for her. She'll enjoy it and it'll help with the ED
16. Lose those extra pounds. It'll help too
17. If you smoke, stop no matter how hard it is
18. Check your prostate
19. Look hard at the foods you're eating
20. Stress and guilt are bad, bad, bad. Just don't do it
21. Try a penis pump

*Use the back of this page to write down your own tools. Remember, not every method will work every time. **So try several of them each time.** Good luck!*

From Michelle:

Almost forgot: I never told you guys what I do for a living. I have two degrees from Baylor University. One is in print media. The other is in marketing.

I retired from the newspaper business several years ago and now make a living writing books under the pen name Charlie Bennett.

The marketing side of me would be remiss if I didn't gift you with a free sample of my work.

Hey, it's what marketers do.

Please enjoy this absolutely free sample of my book **"1001 Little Known Things About Well-Known People.***"*

If you like the free sample and want to read more, the book is available on Amazon.com.

If you're not interested in buying the book, enjoy the free sample anyway.

0001.

You all remember singer and actress Whitney Houston. Her powerful voice sent chills up one's spine, and she was as beautiful as she was talented. You know her work, including the movie *The Bodyguard* and the song *I Will Always Love You*. But did you know she was the most awarded female act of all time? It's true. You can look it up in the 2009 Guinness Book of World Records.

0002.

Jerry Mathers played Beaver Cleaver on *Leave it to Beaver* for a very short time, yet it's still shown somewhere in the world every minute of every day in syndication. You'd think Mr. Mathers must be a rich man from all the residual money he's raking in. But you'd be wrong. Back then they didn't give actors residuals. He doesn't make a penny from them.

0003.

Actor George Reeves played the first *Superman*, in the black and white TV series of the same name in the 1950s. Did you know he committed suicide?

0004.

Actor John Ritter, most famous for his role as Jack Tripper in the ABC sitcom *Three's Company*, was zany, mischievous, and had a great sense of humor. He would likely have had a very long line of choice acting gigs had he not died tragically in 2003. Here's something you didn't know about him: His father was country music legend Tex Ritter.

0005.

Even kids born in the twenty-first century know who John Wayne was. Most well known for his calm speaking voice, tough persona and his rugged portrayal of an American cowboy, he was so much more. He once played football for the University of Southern California and had aspirations of playing professional ball. He injured himself in a bodysurfing accident though, and lost his scholarship. And the rest, as they say, is history.

0006.
Those of you who are fans of 1950s-era Rock 'n' Roll have listened to Buddy Holly's soulful rendition *It Doesn't Matter Anymore.* But we'll bet you didn't know it was written by Paul Anka, who was a friend of Holly's.

0007.
Think you knew all there was to know about former U.S. President Gerald Ford? We'll bet you didn't know he was once the mystery guest on the TV show *What's My Line?*

0008.
Rosanna Arquette (*Desperately Seeking Susan, Pulp Fiction*) is an accomplished American actress and producer. She's also a very distant relative of legendary explorer Meriweather Lewis (of Lewis and Clark fame)

0009.
You'd have to travel the earth and speak to a lot of people to find one who didn't know one of the most famous aliens of all time: Mr. Spock from the *Star Trek* series of television shows and feature films. Leonard Nimoy, of course, played the role. But it wasn't the first time he played an alien. Ask those same people about his previous out-of-this-world role

and very few can identify it. In 1952 he portrayed a Martian named Narab in a movie serial called *Zombies of the Stratosphere.*

0010.
Eliza Dushku (*Buffy the Vampire Slayer, Angel, Tru Calling, True Lies, Bring It On, Wrong Turn*) is a classic beauty and an actress who grew up, literally, on the silver screen. She not only had starring roles in two successful series, but also several box office blockbusters as well. She has an Albanian eagle tattooed on the back of her neck. It's a tribute to her Albanian heritage (on her father's side). She's a citizen of Albania too, by the way.

0011.
American actor Tim *Robbins (Shawshank Redemption, Mystic River, Bull Durham, Dead Man Walking)* is one of film audience's most loved players. He's another kind of player as well. He's a big ice hockey fan and plays in one of New York City's recreational leagues every chance he gets.

0012.
Rock 'n' Roll singer Richie Valens died at the tender age of 17. There isn't a lot of video available of him because he simply didn't live long enough to make a lot of movies or television appearances. He did appear in one movie, though. It was called *Go, Johnny, Go.* He sang his hit *La Bamba.*

0013.
John Travolta is known for the many roles he played in a variety of genre, from *Welcome Back Kotter to Saturday Night Fever* to *Pulp Fiction.* We think he did quite well for a high school drop-out.

0014.

Ralph Waite was an accomplished actor, best known for his role as John Walton Sr., the kind father in *The Waltons* family, as well as a role in *Cool Hand Luke*. As a boy during World War II he wanted very much to help in the war effort. But he was just too young. He had to wait until 1946 to become a United States Marine.

0015.

Chevy Chase was known for his dry wit and pratfalls, and to this day remains an icon in American culture. You've seen some of his movies. Everybody has. Our personal favorite is *Fletch*. Did you know he once wrote for *Mad Magazine*?

0016.

Actress Lauren Graham is best known for her seven year stint as Lorelei on *The Gilmore Girls*. But there is so much more to know about her. For example, did you know she was born in Hawaii and lived for several years in Japan?

0017.

Actor Ben Affleck's natural good looks and boyish charm easily make him a fan favorite on the silver screen. But there's much more to the *Good Will Hunting* and *Pearl Harbor* actor than just a pretty face. When he was a teenager he learned to speak Spanish and filmed a children's television show in Mexico.

0018.

British actress Kate Beckinsale (born Kathrin Romary Beckinsale in 1973) has a long and impressive list of film credits. They include *Brokedown Palace, Pearl*

Harbor, *Serendipity*, *The Aviator* and *Click*. But her screen debut occurred much earlier. She first appeared on television at age four, on an episode of *This is Your Life*.

0019.
Olympic swimmer Michael Phelps has won more medals than any other athlete in any Olympic games. Going into the 2016 Olympic Games in Rio, he had an astonishing 23 Olympic medals. Not bad for a guy who has AD/HD.

0020.
Sylvester Stallone (*Rocky, The Expendables, Rambo*) has always played a tough guy on the silver screen. So you'd be forgiven if you thought he was long on muscle, short on brains. Not true at all. Sly was a graduate from the University of Miami and wrote or co-wrote many of his films.

0021.
For millennials, former President Dwight D. Eisenhower is just a name in a history book. All his accomplishments have been largely forgotten. But here's a little tidbit which might make him a bit more relatable: He was the very first president to appear on national television.

0022.
Love him or hate him, Texas Senator Ted Cruz is a powerful force in American politics. He wasn't born Ted, or even Theodore. He was born Rafael Edward Cruz. Where in heck did "Ted" come from?

0023.
Lauren Cohan is arguably the prettiest zombie killer
we know. She made her bones (get it?) on the AMC
series *The Walking Dead*, and frequently guest stars
on the hit *Supernatural* as well. Did you know that in
real life she speaks with a heavy British accent?
That's because although she was born in New Jersey,
she moved to England when she was a year old.

0024.
Johnny Cash and his music have made a resurgence of
late, and the late country singer is almost as well
known today as he was in his heyday. We've all heard
his song *A Boy Named Sue*. But I'll bet you didn't
know the song was written by a cartoonist.
Specifically, the legendary cartoonist for *Playboy*
magazine Shel Silverstein.

0025.
Big Bang Theory has become one of the best loved
sitcoms in history, thanks in no small part to Jim
Parsons, who plays Sheldon Cooper on the show. Jim
is an ancestor of the famous French architect Louis-
Francois Trouard.

0026.
O'Shea Jackson Sr., known professionally as Ice
Cube, is many things. An accomplished actor, a
talented hip hop singer, a record producer, songwriter
and producer. He's obviously pretty darned smart,
which is why it only took him one year to obtain his
degree from the Phoenix Institute of Technology. In
architecture, of all things.

0027.
Astronaut Buzz Aldrin wasn't just known for his walk upon the lunar surface. He was known among his peers for his sense of humor, his love for playing pranks, and his ability to turn a phrase. He used to brag that he was the "first man to piss his pants on the moon."

0028.
Jay Z (born Shawn Carter) is one of the most successful rappers in history. But it hasn't always been smooth sailing. He's been shot three times.

0029.
Audrey Drake Graham is known professionally as Drake, and is a successful rapper and actor, record producer and songwriter.   Did you know he's Canadian and spent most of his childhood in Toronto?

0030.
President Gerald Ford was known for his lack of grace, and even made fun of his own clumsiness. He occasionally suffered a vocal miscue as well. He once was quoted as saying, "I love baseball. I watch a lot of it on the radio."

0031.
Love him or hate him, Barack Obama is an interesting man. That cannot be disputed. One of the people he wanted to impress the most in his life was his grandmother, Madelyn Dunham. And she was indeed proud of him, but never got to see him elected president. She died just two days before the election in 2008.

0032.
Elizabeth Taylor was one of Hollywood's best loved actresses. Did you know she made her television debut on a soap opera? It's true. *General Hospital*, in 1981.

0033.
Kelly Bishop played Lorelei Gilmore's sometimes unlikeable mother Emily in *The Gilmore Girls*. In real life she is personable and sweet-tempered, a testament to her impressive acting abilities. Did you know she was once a ballet dancer, and was good enough to do it professionally?

0034.
Paul Edward Giamatti (*Big Fat Liar, Straight Outa Compton, Downton Abbey*), is one of Hollywood's most successful character actors. But there are a few things you didn't know about him. For example, did you know out of his 94 TV and movie roles, he's only been nominated for one Oscar (for *Cinderella Man*)?

0035.
Keiko Agena is a Japanese-American actress best known for her portrayal as Lane in the long-running series The Gilmore Girls. She played a teenage girl and best friend of second lead (and also teenage girl) Rory Gilmore. But Agena wasn't a teenager. She was 27 when the series started, a full eleven years older than Alexis Bledel, who played Rory.

0036.
Italian and American actress Sophia Loren had other ties to history besides the silver screen. She was also the godmother to Benito Mussolini's grandson.

0037.
Steven Yeun was born in Korea but raised in America. He's best known for his portrayal as Glenn Rhee in the hit series *Walking Dead*. If anyone on the show can understand the physiological makeup of a zombie it would be Steven. He has a degree in psychology with a concentration in neuroscience.

0038.
Jared Padalecki is perhaps best known for his role as Sam Winchester on *Supernatural*. If you've wondered about his last name, it's Polish. But there's much more running through Jared's blood. He can also trace his ancestry to Germany, Scotland, England and France.

0039.
He's been dead for generations, but Mark Twain continues to be one of the world's best loved authors. You thought you already knew everything about the man. But did you know he was the very first writer to present a typewritten manuscript to his publisher?

0040.
Actor Kevin Bacon (*Footloose, JFK, A Few Good Men, Apollo 13, Mystic River*) took preparation for a role to a whole new level. When preparing for his role in Footloose, he felt he needed a refresher course in how teenagers interacted with one another. So he went undercover, as a high school student, to observe them. The only reason he got away with it was because of his youthful appearance and the fact he was relatively unknown then.

0041.

Anyone who's ever watched reruns of the old *Brady Bunch* TV show remember Alice the maid (her last name on the show was Nelson, although that was never revealed). Her real name was Ann B. Davis. Did you know she had an identical twin sister?

0042.

Actress Shirley Temple was America's little sweetheart for many years. Everybody knows that. Everybody also knows she was a United States ambassador for many years as well. But very few people know she was a successful adult actress. It's true. She even starred opposite John Wayne in the movie classic *She Wore a Yellow Ribbon.*

0043.

Allyson Felix is a U.S. sprinter who has racked up an impressive number of Olympic medals. Nine, to be exact. She weighed 125 pounds in high school, yet her legs were so strong she dead-lifted 270 pounds. Her nickname back then was "Chicken Legs."

0044.

Bob Crane was the affable Captain Hogan in the TV series *Hogan's Heroes.* The popular series can still be seen around the world in syndication even today. Did you know Bob Crane was murdered, supposedly by a kinky sex partner?

0045.

American President Richard Nixon fought hard to maintain a stalwart personal image, even as the Watergate scandal tore down his presidency. He once pleaded with good friend and Secretary of State Henry

Kissinger, "Henry, promise me you won't tell them I cried."

0046.
Those of you who are fans of 1950s-era Rock 'n' Roll are likely fans of Buddy Holly as well. Did you know his real name wasn't Holly but Holley? It's true. The name was misspelled on his first record contract. Instead of making waves and invalidating the contract, he just decided to use it as a stage name.

0047.
Thomas Jeffrey (Tom) Hanks has acted in and produced films which have grossed nearly five billion dollars, making him one of the biggest moneymakers in film history. As a child he moved quite often. By the time he was ten years of age he'd already lived in ten different houses.

0048.
One of veteran actor Harrison Ford's most memorable roles was that of Indiana Jones, kind of a super hero/adventurer/boy scout type. That characterization isn't very far off the mark. As a young man he was very active in boy scouts, achieving the second highest award of "Life Scout."

0049.
Martin Sheen (born Ramón Antonio Gerardo Estévez) is an accomplished actor and director (*Badlands*, *Apocalypse Now*, *Gettysburg*, *The West Wing*). When he was born in Dayton, Ohio back in 1940, his left arm was crushed by a doctor's forceps. To this very day, he has limited lateral movement in that arm, which is three inches shorter than his right arm.

0050.

Dustin Hoffman is an accomplished actor who has left in mark in many memorable roles. Who can forget *Rain Man* and *The Graduate*? Hoffman's rugged good looks made him a favorite among the ladies especially. But not everyone shared that opinion. When he was young and announced he wanted to go into acting, his Aunt Pearl announced, "You can't be an actor. You're not good looking enough."

0051.

This whole Kardashian thing… Some love them and some can't stand them. Many just think the world would be a better place if they'd never been "discovered." That almost was the case, by the way. Their father Robert Kardashian was a relatively unknown attorney until O.J. Simpson's murder case put him in the national spotlight. It was only then the media noticed he had some attractive daughters. In other words, you can blame O.J. for the whole Kardashian phenomenon.

0052.

American actress Cybill Shepard *(The Last Picture Show, The Heartbreak Kid, Taxi Driver, Moonlighting)* was also a successful fashion model and beauty queen. She was named after Cy, her grandfather, and Bill, her dad.

0053.

Peyton Manning played eighteen years as quarterback for the Indianapolis Colts and Denver Broncos. He's considered one of the best quarterbacks of all time. Maybe it's because it's in his blood. His father, Archie Manning, played quarterback for the New Orleans Saints for many years.

0054.

American actor Tom Cruise (*Taps, Risky Business, Mission: Impossible, Top Gun*) has been one of Hollywood's biggest success stories for a very long time. But things weren't always easy for him. He grew up in a very abusive environment, being constantly beaten by his father. He later called his father a "bully and a coward."

0055.

Annabella Avery Thorne is known professionally as Bella Thorne. She's one of television's rising young stars, with roles in *Shake it Up, My Own Worst Enemy*, and *Blended*. She's a fair skinned, red headed beauty. She doesn't look it, but she's part Cuban.

0056.

Most of you remember Jerry Lewis as the man who emceed the Muscular Dystrophy telethon for so many years. Those who are older will remember his movies with Dean Martin. You millennials may not remember him at all. Here's something none of you knew: he was once nominated for a Nobel Prize.

0057.

Cordozar Calvin Broadus, Jr. recently sold his thirty six millionth album. What? You don't know who Cordozar Calvin Broadus, Jr. is? Well, perhaps you know him by his other name: Snoop Dogg. Not bad for a guy with a funny name.

0058.

Alexis Bledel is an American actress who's had several successful roles. She's best known, though, for her portrayal as Rory in *The Gilmore Girls*. Her first language was Spanish, and she didn't even learn

English until she started grade school. Despite her striking blue eyes and fair skin, she considers herself Hispanic.

0059.
American actress Sarah Anne Wayne Callies is best known for her role as Lori Grimes in the hit show *Walking Dead*. Her character in the show was killed. Did you know that was her idea? She convinced the writers and producers to kill her character to remain true to the print version of the story.

Printed in Great Britain
by Amazon

59276639R00129